Living with an Acquired Brain Injury

A Practical Life Skills Workbook

Living with an
Acquired Brain Injury

A Practical Life Skills Workbook

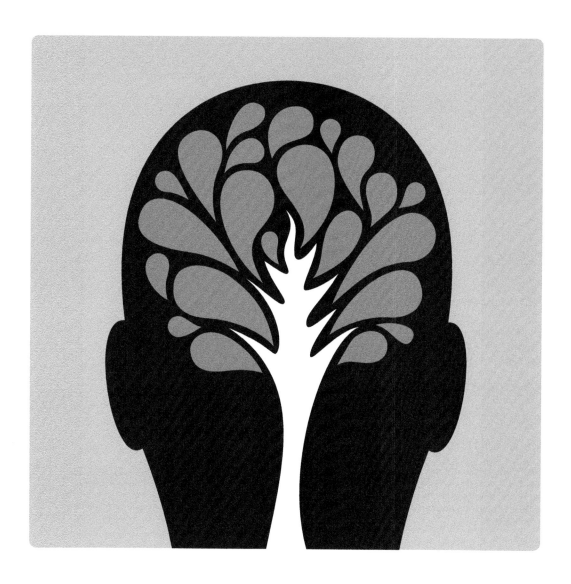

Nicholas Hedley

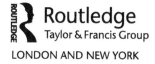

Routledge
Taylor & Francis Group

LONDON AND NEW YORK

Supplementary Resources Disclaimer

Additional resources were previously made available for this title on CD. However, as CD has become a less accessible format, all resources have been moved to a more convenient online download option.

You can find these resources available here: http://resourcecentre.routledge.com/books/9780863888106

Please note: Where this title mentions the associated disc, please use the downloadable resources instead.

First published 2011 by Speechmark Publishing Ltd.

Published 2017 by Routledge
2 Park Square, Milton Park, Abingdon, Oxon OX14 4RN
711 Third Avenue, New York, NY 10017, USA

Routledge is an imprint of the Taylor & Francis Group, an informa business

Printed and bound by CPI Group (UK) Ltd, Croydon, CR0 4YY

British Library Cataloguing in Publication Data

ISBN: 9780863888106 (pbk)

Contents

Introduction

Living with an Acquired Brain Injury is designed for people who have recovered well enough from brain injury to prepare for a return to independent living. Although all brain injuries are different, there is a common pattern of stages amongst the majority of acquired brain injury survivors. They are:

1 Acquired Brain Injury.

2 Immediately post injury, hospital, intensive care, in-depth monitoring, support and possibly surgery.

3 When the patient no longer needs intensive care or high dependency support they will remain in hospital. Brain injury affects many in some physical, psychological and cognitive way. In-hospital rehabilitation is necessary for the patient to function adequately beyond the hospital doors.

4 Once the hospital time ends, return home.

Because of the varying degrees of brain injury, the severity of the injury plays a part. It should be remembered that each brain injury is unique in its post brain injury symptoms. The following symptoms are general and not everyone experiences all of them. However, they are considered characteristic of post brain injury:

- A physical disability
- Headaches
- Fatigue
- Short-term memory issues
- Cognitive problems
- Attention and concentration difficulties
- Speed of information processing
- Often, a brain injury can result in epilepsy.

Bearing this in mind, some individuals who have suffered a brain injury may be unable to reach the stage this book aims to aid in achieving. It is very important never to rush sufferers of a brain injury.

For many people this workbook will represent a milestone in the journey towards living independently. The activities included will allow you to practise and develop your knowledge of and skills for some everyday tasks, which can initially appear daunting.

It has been designed to be a very accessible and easy to read resource, taking learning styles after brain injury into account. This workbook can be completed at the pace that best suits *you*.

Exercises and tips included in the book cover:

- Budgeting: This is perhaps the most important skill required in a return to independent life.

- Reading and understanding bill terminology: In order to budget effectively you must be able to understand the terminology used in your bills.

- Route orientation: When out of the house, particularly after acquiring brain injury, orientating your way around can be difficult and even intimidating, often due to short term memory issues. Many people with an acquired brain injury also have visual spatial awareness problems. Often places familiar in the past can now seem unfamiliar. Learning to find your way around safely is a very important skill.

- Form filling: To access many things in life, you will need to fill in forms. There are rules involved in form filling, and with a little practice and guidance, you can master this skill.

- Planning a night's entertainment: Skills involved in this go beyond the TV remote control, or a night at the pub and involve planning a night out.

The book as a whole, including the activities, is designed to be completed over a period of ten weeks. This is not as intensive as it may sound. The intended 'easy going' approach recommended is:

- Week 1: Spend 45 minutes of one day in week 2 working on a topic.

- Week 2: Spend 45 minutes of one day in week 2 working on the same topic as week 1 to aid in the consolidation of memory for the topic.

This will continue for each topic. The topics are presented in a specific order in the book intentionally, and it is recommended that you follow this. Some topics are more interesting than others due to the bureaucratic nature of some of the important skills, which you will need in life.

A recommended timetable for completing the workbook follows; however, if you feel you are able to work through more of the book in one sitting, or prefer to work at a faster or slower rate, then you can do so. It is important to work at a pace that suits *you*.

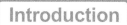
Workbook completion timetable

Week	Activities	Time
1	Budgeting	45 minutes
2	Budgeting	45 minutes
3	Reading and understanding bill terminology	45 minutes
4	Reading and understanding bill terminology	45 minutes
5	Route orientation	45 minutes
6	Route orientation	45 minutes
7	Form filling	45 minutes
8	Form filling	45 minutes
9	Planning a night's entertainment	45 minutes
10	Planning a night's entertainment	45 minutes

Part A: Activities

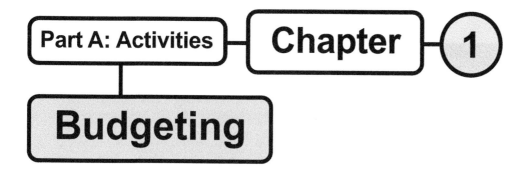

Part A: Activities — Chapter — 1

Budgeting

Effective budgeting is perhaps the most important practical life skill presented in this book, and organising and planning your finances is an essential part of life.

The amount of money you have in the bank is called a bank 'balance'. It is important to keep your bank account 'balanced'. The amount of money coming out of your bank account cannot be more than the amount of money going in. If you do overspend and you do not have enough money in your account you will become overdrawn. If this happens, the bank will charge you a fee.

You may be paid weekly or monthly, depending on your circumstances. If you spend too much at the beginning of the week or month, you may not have enough money remaining to pay for essentials. A useful task is to write down a list of the things that you spend money on. Then rewrite the list in order of importance, including expenditure such as rent, food and utility bills. You will probably find that these expenditures come at the top, while the least important will be at the bottom of the list. This is prioritising. Important necessity expenditure like food and rent are the highest priority. Crisps and confectionary are a good example of non-necessity expenditure. They are nice, but we can live without them.

Monetary calculation is necessary for successful budgeting; a calculator is recommended to make managing, planning and organising your finances easier.

Budgeting table

A budgeting table is an organised way to keep track of your finances. An average person's budgeting table should be quite simple and easy to use. An example table follows.

Payment taken Payment received Title	Money in	Money out	Resulting bank account balance

A blank template provided at the end of the book can be photocopied. You may find this useful. You can fill in the categories yourself. If you wish to add more categories or columns, you can draw your own.

It is advisable to try to save a certain amount of money per week or month. This will continue to grow. Ultimately this has the bonus of covering unexpected bills or it could be used to save for something more expensive, such as a holiday. If circumstances change, allowances and priorities may also need to change. An example could be someone who loses their job. Some items they used to buy before may now be non-essential, so these things may be reduced in quantity. Alternatively you may actually remove these items altogether.

Practise your budgeting skills by completing the budgeting activities in this workbook. In the first budgeting task, you will learn to prioritise expenditure, ie what is essential and what is non-essential.

Time to get started…

Routledge
Taylor & Francis Group

Prioritising activities

Prioritising activity 1

Jack is a taxi driver.

He is married with two children.

He is buying his home and pays a mortgage.

His hobby is fishing.

Using the expenses sheet that follows, complete the budget sheet for Jack. Prioritise his expenditure:

- Number 1 will be the most essential.
- Number 15 will be the least essential.

Routledge
Taylor & Francis Group

Taxi driver Jack's expenses

- Council tax

- Expenditure for family (clothes etc)

- Mortgage

- Garage fees for repairs to car

- CDs for in-car CD player

- Petrol

- Holiday

- Food and groceries

- New fishing equipment

- Fuel bills, gas and electricity

- Monthly motoring magazine

- Phone bill

- Repayment of personal loan

- Leisure (cinema, restaurants)

- Water rates

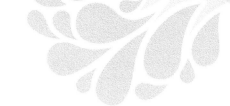

Taxi driver Jack's budget sheet

1

2

3

4

5

6

7

8

9

10

11

12

13

14

15

R Routledge Taylor & Francis Group   Living with an Acquired Brain Injury   11

Prioritising activity 2

Jane, Denise and Karen are three nurses. They are single and share a flat.

They all work at the same hospital and they all own their own cars.

They want to go on holiday together and must prioritise their spending to save enough money to pay for their holiday.

Plan a budget for the nurses. They spend too much. If they want their holiday they must economise.

Using the budget sheet write down their priorities. Reduce their expenditure by cutting down on things they do not need.

Routledge Taylor & Francis Group

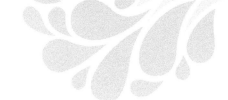

Nurses' expenses

- Shoes
- Car tyres
- Parties
- Rent
- Clubbing
- Phone bill
- Gown hire
- Karen's archery club
- Electricity
- Jane's cookery classes
- Council tax
- Food
- Petrol
- Denise's flying lessons
- Wine making kit

Nurses' budget sheet

1

2

3

4

5

6

7

8

9

10

11

12

13

14

15

Routledge
Taylor & Francis Group

Prioritising activity 3

Brian is 37, and has lost his job. He now receives jobseeker's allowance.

He is single and lives in a rented flat. He receives housing and council tax benefit. He owns a car.

Although he has some savings he must budget more carefully until he finds another job.

Prioritise Brian's spending. What can he do without until he finds employment, so that he does not have to spend all of his savings?

Brian's expenses

- Weekly football magazine

- Petrol

- Toiletries

- Night out (cinema, pub)

- Clothing

- Take-away food

- Household cleaning products

- Gas and electricity

- Food

- Newspapers

- Paint balling sessions

- Holidays

- Tickets for football match

Brian's budget sheet

1

2

3

4

5

6

7

8

9

10

11

12

13

14

15

Routledge
Taylor & Francis Group

Numerical calculation activities

Numerical calculation activity 1

Mrs Higgins is a school teacher and has two young children. She is a single parent.

She owns a car and earns £400 a week.
She receives a child benefit of £31 per week.

She pays a mortgage.

Mrs Higgins wants to take her children on holiday.

On the budget sheet provided, write down Mrs Higgins' priority spending. Cut down on the things that she can do without so that she has money left at the end of the week to save for her holiday.

Routledge
Taylor & Francis Group

Mrs Higgins' weekly expenses

• Cinema	£20.00
• Food	£70.00
• Lottery	£5.00
• Petrol	£30.00
• Childcare	£40.00
• Magazines	£10.00
• Council tax	£10.00
• Clothes	£25.00
• Plants	£15.00
• Mortgage	£105.00
• Gas and electric	£30.00
• Mobile phone bill	£25.00

Total = £385.00

Routledge
Taylor & Francis Group

Living with an Acquired Brain Injury

Mrs Higgins' budget sheet

Incoming:

Total =	

Outgoing:

Total =	

Living with an Acquired Brain Injury

Routledge
Taylor & Francis Group

Numerical calculation activity 2

Kevin is single and lives in a rented flat.

He owns a car and earns £350 a week.

He would like to buy a new car.

How can Kevin reduce his expenditure?

Make a budget sheet for Kevin. Prioritise his spending so that he can save enough to buy a new car.

Remove non-essential spending and see how much Kevin can save each week towards his new car.

Kevin's weekly expenses

- CDs   £8.00
- Gym session   £10.00
- Food   £50.00
- Cinema and pub   £30.00
- Petrol   £36.00
- Phone bill   £15.00
- Electricity   £14.00
- Magazines   £8.00
- Rent and council tax   £125.00
- Car insurance   £5.00
- Life insurance policy   £4.00

Total = £305.00

Routledge
Taylor & Francis Group

Kevin's budget sheet

Incoming:

Total =	

Outgoing:

Total =	

Numerical calculation activity 3

Kate is 19 years old and is unemployed.

She lives with her parents.

She claims a jobseeker's allowance of £47.95 per week.

She is spending more money than she has coming in.

Plan a weekly budget sheet for Kate. Prioritise her spending so that she does not overspend.

What does she need to spend money on, and what can she do without until she finds a job?

Routledge
Taylor & Francis Group

Kate's weekly expenses

• Make-up	£6.00
• Cinema	£10.00
• Clothes	£20.00
• Board money to parents	£15.00
• Fashion magazine	£5.00
• Mobile phone	£5.00
• Bus fares	£7.00
	Total = £68.00

Routledge
Taylor & Francis Group

Kate's budget sheet

Incoming:

Total =

Outgoing:

Total =

Routledge
Taylor & Francis Group

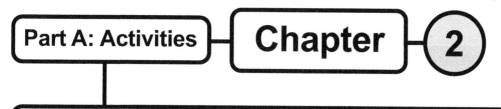

Reading and understanding bill terminology

The services we receive that we often take for granted must be paid for. When we have to pay for these services, we are sent a bill. This is a document stating how much we need to pay, and how much of the service we have used. Examples of a bill are your water or phone bill.

Bill terminology is the specific words and phrases commonly used in the bills that you will receive. In order to budget independently and effectively, you will need to understand this terminology. Reading and understanding the terminology of bills is another vital skill necessary for living independently. Effectively this topic goes hand-in-hand with budgeting, as it is necessary to understand the bills that you will receive, so that you may manage your money effectively.

The specific terminology used in bills will differ from bill to bill. The terminology used in a water bill will not be used in your phone bill, and the same goes for all combinations of bills.

Despite this, you will notice some similar terms used in all bills, 'account number' is one such term. Each party or company that you receive a bill from will hold your details on their computers. To save them time in finding your details should you ever need to contact them, they can just enter your account number into their computer and your details (address and so on), will come up on their computer monitor. It is very important to remember that every party, organisation or company who send you bills, all have their own individual account number for you. For example, your council tax account number will not be the same as your mobile phone account number.

A common charge on bills is VAT (value added tax). This is a tax charged on most business transactions.

Some of the activities in this chapter require you to use numerical calculation. Your number skills are not being tested here, just your ability to understand the bill terminology questions.

One of the most important 'bills' you will receive, which is not a request for payment, is your bank statement. Reading and understanding this particular 'bill' is a vital part of budgeting (the first topic covered in this workbook). This shows you the activity in your bank account, for example, the money being paid into your account (wages or benefits), as well as the money being taken out of your account (cash taken from ATM machines, direct debits and standing orders).

Bill 1: Bank statement

Bank statement terminology

- Bank statement: A bank statement is a financial record of the activity in your bank account.

- Account number: This is the number of your account, and the bank's method for identifying you and your personal details.

- Sort code: This is a number that is assigned to a branch of a bank for the bank's own purposes. Banks use sort codes as it is easier than writing out the full address of the branch out and it tells customers which branch of the particular bank they are in. In the following example, it is the Vivelchester branch of Delta Bank.

- Bank balance: The amount of money you have in your account is called your bank balance.

- Deposit: An amount of money paid into your bank account. This can also come under the heading 'paid in'.

- ATM (automated teller machine): A cash machine.

- Direct debit: This is a regular payment that you allow to be taken from your bank account to pay for a service, for example, a phone or electricity bill.

- Standing order: This term refers to money that you regularly pay out to a company. This is similar to a direct debit, but with a standing order you are paying out, as opposed to giving someone else permission to take money.

Routledge
Taylor & Francis Group

Example bank statement

Delta Bank

Ms Jane Smith
113 Potterton Way
Yorksdale
Vivelchester
NE17 6ST

Account Number: 24646798
Sort Code: 12-34-56

1 September 2009

Date	Details	Withdrawn	Paid in	Balance
2009	BROUGHT FORWARD			72.74
03 Aug	Rita's Music Store Card Transaction	22.00		50.74
05 Aug	Bankleton ATM	30.00		20.74
10 Aug	Bank Giro Credit REF00332DWP DLA		95.00	115.74
05 Aug	Vivelchester Food Mart	27.53		88.21
16 Aug	Love 2 Talk Mobile Phone direct debit	16.00		72.21
20 Aug	This Travel shop card transaction	18.50		53.71
23 Aug	Branch pay-in (**cheque**)		65.00	118.71
30 Aug	Mr & Mrs C Doddson **standing order**	60.00		58.71
31 Aug	Blue Moon Chemist Card Transaction	7.23		51.48

Delta Bank

Activity 1 – Bank statement terminology

Write the answers in the boxes provided.

1 A document giving you information about your bank account.

2 Funds paid into your bank account.

3 Allowing a debit as regular payment to a company for a service provided, eg a phone bill.

4 Funds taken out of your bank account.

5 Allowing your bank to pay money from your account on a regular basis to an external party.

6 How much money you have in your account.

7 Your personal number.

8 Number of a particular branch.

Routledge
Taylor & Francis Group

Activity 2 – Bank statement terminology

Calculate answers to the questions and write them in the boxes provided.

1 What is the total of the two lowest withdrawals from 03/08/09 to 31/08/09?

£ _____

2 What was the total amount of money paid into Ms Smith's account?

£ _____

3 What is the total amount of money withdrawn from a cash machine from 03/08/09 to 31/08/09?

£ _____

4 How many times did Ms Smith use her debit card from 03/08/09 to 31/08/09?

_____ times

5 Look at the end balance on Ms Smith's bank statement. Is her account in credit or debit?

_____

6 How much disability living allowance (DLA) was paid into her account between 03/08/09 and 31/08/09?

£ _____

7 How much money was withdrawn from Ms Smith's bank account between 03/08/09 and 31/08/09?

£ _____

8 How many times was money taken out of Ms Smith's bank account in the period of time covered by the statement?

_____ times

R Routledge Taylor & Francis Group   Living with an Acquired Brain Injury   31

Bill 2: Council tax bill

Council tax is used to pay for public services. These include council services, fire and rescue and the police.

Council tax bill terminology

- Date of issue: The date that the bill was written or sent.

- Details of charge: The service that you are being charged for, for example, fire and rescue, or the police.

- Reference number: Unique to your bill. As with your bank account number, this number will need to be given when you communicate with the senders of the bill.

- Property reference: The number that the council have given your particular house. Many flats have the same door number and street name, so this is how the council identify you, your property and your account with them.

- Charge for period: The dates and length of time that your bill covers.

- Annual: Once a year.

- Amount due: The amount of council tax that you owe.

- Instalments: A method of paying. If you cannot afford to pay all the bill at once, you can split the cost into instalments, and pay monthly, for example.

- Band: All homes are given a council tax valuation band. The band is based on the value of your home. A different amount of council tax is charged for each band. For example, the owner of a lower cost property (a house in Band A), would pay less council tax than the owner of a more expensive house in Band H.

R Routledge
Taylor & Francis Group

Example council tax bill

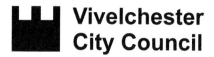 **Vivelchester City Council**

Council Tax Demand Note

Email: council.tax@Vivelchester.gov.uk
www.vivelchester.gov.uk/counciltax

Address any enquiries to

COUNCIL TAX,
P.O.BOX 1 UP
VIVELCHESTER
NE49 7PQ

or telephone 0845 222 3249
8:00am-6:00pm Monday to Friday.

To   43664615
John Smith
113 Potterton Way
Yorksdale
Vivelchester NE17 6ST

Date of Issue   **17-Mar-2010**
Property Reference   **160719**

Reference Number: 2169 9905 339. Reason for Bill: Annual

This is your Council Tax bill; details of how this bill has been calculated as well as payments due are shown in the box below. The above property is shown in the Local Validation List as BAND A property.

Details of Charge	Amount (£)	Change (%)
Vivelchester City Council	865.26	3.9
Vivelchester Fire and Rescue	47.74	2.4
Vivelchester Police Authority	52.18	4.9
Total Charge	965.18	

	(£)
Charge for Period Band A 01-April-2009 to 31-March-2010	965.18
Amount Due	**965.18**

Activity – Council tax bill terminology

Write the answers in the boxes provided.

1 Date the bill was issued.

2 Details of how the money from your council tax is spent.

3 The personal number you will need if you contact the council about your bill.

4 The dates you are being billed for.

5 Bill paid once a year.

6 The amount of council tax you must pay now.

7 Name another way that you could pay your council tax so you would not have to pay in one large amount.

8 Which service receives the least amount of council tax funds?

Routledge
Taylor & Francis Group

Bill 3: Home phone bill

Home phone bill terminology

- Length of calls: How long each call lasted.

- Cost of calls: How much each call costs. Calls to mobile phones or abroad will cost more than a local call.

- Type of call: The category of call, eg weekend, evening, free calls.

- Total cost of calls: This can be the total cost of all calls together, or the total cost of calls that fall under a particular category, ie weekend and evenings, free calls. To find out the full total cost of all calls, add together the £ numerical value of each category of call.

- VAT: A tax charged on most business transactions.

- Brought Forward: Money that you had left over after the last bill.

- Benefits: Included in the example that follows, an additional option to add to your phone price plan which enables you to get calls at a discount rate. The 'friends together option 1', printed near the top of the bill, is the name of the benefit option chosen for this original price plan. This particular benefit means that calls made to friends are charged at a discount rate, so costs you less. Different bills and price plans will have different names for this special type of offer.

Ultimately it is impossible to list all bill terminology, as there are so many different kinds of bills for different services or other purchase transactions. If you are in doubt over any part of your bill, it is always advisable to phone the company or person who sent the bill to discuss anything that is unclear.

Example home phone bill

Account Number: B47G8855   Bill Number: ROO4 DK   Number: 0191 5724579

Bill Date: 30 Mar 10   Debit balance   £28.62

Friends Together Option 1

Statement for: 0191 5724579

Bill Period 31st Dec 2009-30 Mar 2010

DEBIT BALANCE: £28.62

Cost of Calls:	£15.69
Your Benefits:	-£1.29
Rental Charges:	£91.15
VAT:	£20.52
Total this period:	£126.07
Brought Forward:	£2.55
Payments:	£100.00
Debit Balance:	£28.62

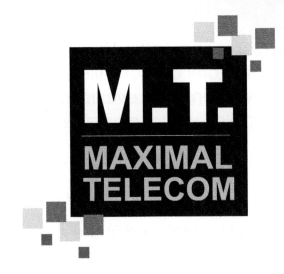

Type of call	Total number of calls	Total duration	Cost (£)
Free calls	3	0000:30:21	0.00
Daytime	115	0004:19:22	14.915
Evenings and Weekends	18	0002:00:25	0.771

Routledge
Taylor & Francis Group

Activity – Home phone bill terminology

These questions are about the phone bill you have been given. In the cost of calls summary:

1 How many free calls were made?

2 How long did they last?

3 How much did they cost?

4 How many daytime calls were made?

5 How long did they last?

6 How much did they cost?

7 How many evening and weekend calls were made?

8 How long did they last?

9 How much did they cost?

10 What was the total cost of calls?

11 How much were the benefits?

12 How much were the rental charges?

13 How much was brought forward?

14 How much VAT was added to the bill?

15 How much do you have to pay Maximal Telecom? £

Routledge
Taylor & Francis Group

Bill 4: Mobile phone bill

Mobile phone bill terminology

- Account number: You will be getting to know this now. However, each account number you have will be different for each bill. The number will never be the same from one company to the next.

- Service charge: The fixed amount your mobile phone service charges you for its price plan.

- VAT: A tax charged on most business transactions.

- Price plan: This is the option that you chose for your phone service provider. Deltaphone is the phone service provider in the mobile phone bill provided as an example. For example, in your price plan you may get 20 free texts per month and 40 minutes of free calls to other mobile phone numbers. This kind of price plan with benefits is common among mobile phone service providers, as they want your custom.

- Direct debit: This is a regular payment taken directly out of your bank account.

- Insurance: Your phone service provider will offer you the chance to pay regular instalments, combined with your monthly bill, to cover the cost of replacing your phone if it is stolen, lost or damaged. Check what kinds of damage or loss your phone insurance covers, as some insurance offers more cover than others. For example, some insurance may not cover loss.

Example mobile phone bill

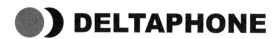

DELTAPHONE

www.deltaphone.co.uk
Give us a call on
08700 223553
email us at
customer.care@deltaphone.co.uk

Account number: 234567890123777
Invoice number: 2345678901

Date: 6th August 2008

J. SMITH
RUDDACK HOUSE
MANCHESTER
NE4 7QP

YOUR PRICE PLAN

**Anytime 125 mins +
Deltaphone megachat + 250 texts
(18 Anytime 125 STC + 250 texts)**

**250 inclusive minutes
to use this month**

**125 rolled over from your
last bill plus 125 in your
price plan**

QUICK BREAKDOWN
For 07911122233

SERVICE CHARGES

18 Anytime 125 STC
+ 250 texts =   £17.02

Video Calling =   £0.00

Cover me Insurance =   £6.95 VAT EXEMPT

USAGE CHARGES up to 29 Jul

Calls =   £0.55

Picture Messaging =   £1.53

TOTAL BEFORE VAT = £26.05

VAT ON THIS BILL =   £3.34

TOTAL =   **£29.39**

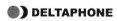

DELTAPHONE

Activity – Mobile phone bill terminology

Write the answers in the boxes provided.

1 Number you must quote when making enquiries about your bill.

2 Fixed cost for your telephone line and any optional equipment.

3 Number the bill is made out to.

4 Tax added to your bill.

5 The personal plan you chose for your phone.

6 Bill paid directly from your bank.

7 Charges made for your calls.

8 Money you pay to cover loss or damage to your phone.

Routledge
Taylor & Francis Group

Bill 5: Water bill

Example water bill

 Vivel Water

| CUSTOMER REFERENCE: 973999020044 |
| BILL NUMBER: 891 |

27th March 2008

J. Smith
7 Houghton Road
Vivelchester
VE3 2XY

Property Address:
J. Smith, 7 Houghton Road
Vivelchester, VE3 2XY

Fixed Charge Period: 01/01/08 to 31/03/08

| Meter Number | Meter Size | Reading Dates | | Reading | | Usage Cubic Metre (M3) |
		Present	Previous	Present	Previous	
97M913920	15	18.03.2008	18.12.2007	1765	1708	57

Balance of last bill issued 24.12.2007	£ 58.23
Sum of payments received (see below)	£ 76.00CR
Sum of other adjustments	£ 00.00
Balance brought forward	**£ 17.77CR**

WATER CHARGES

Fixed @ £28.80 per year	£ 7.20
Usage 28 @ 85.39p per cubic metre	£ 23.91
Usage IS SUBJECT TO A LIMIT OF 28 M3	

SEWERAGE CHARGES

Please see over for details of Surface Water Drainage Rebates

Usage 29 @ 81.61p per cubic metre	£ 23.67
Fixed @ £64.20 per year	£ 16.05
Usage IS SUBJECT TO A LIMIT OF 29 M3	
Total charge for the above period	**£ 70.83**

Total Bill Amount	**£ 17.77CR**

BUDGET ACCOUNT – THIS BILL IS FOR INFORMATION ONLY. PLEASE CONTINUE TO PAY THE AGREED MONTHLY AMOUNT

Payments received with thanks (since last bill)

Date	Amount (£)
25.03.2008	5.00
07.03.2008	5.00
27.02.2008	10.00

R Routledge
Taylor & Francis Group

Activity – Water bill terminology

1 Number you must quote when making a payment.

2 The date the bill was issued.

3 Money brought forward from last bill.

4 Money already paid if you pay your bill weekly.

5 The amount of water you have used and how much it costs.

6 What else is included in your water bill which you must pay for?

7 How is the water that you use measured?

8 Why does it say on this bill 'THIS BILL IS FOR INFORMATION ONLY?'

9 How many cubic metres of water have been used?

10 Write down the reading dates.

Activity – Water bill terminology cont'd

11 What was the date of the previous bill issued?

12 What was the balance brought forward from the previous bill?

13 How much does one cubic metre of water cost?

14 What is the total amount for the bill?

15 How many instalments have been paid?

16 What is the total of the money paid in instalments?

17 What is the issue date of this bill?

18 What is the amount the water charges are fixed at per year?

19 What is the amount the sewerage charges are fixed at per year?

20 Write down the meter number and the meter size.

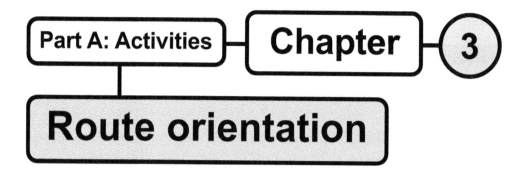

Route orientation

How would you orientate yourself around an unfamiliar place? Wandering around the area of your destination and hoping for the best is certainly not recommended, as you could get lost.

Another way of finding the route to a place that you have never been could be to ask strangers for directions. However, sometimes other people do not know, or could mistakenly give you incorrect directions or very complicated directions, which you may find hard to remember. Therefore, this is an unreliable method of route orientation and it is better to have a more definite knowledge of exactly where you are going. What is usually essential is the use of an external resource, for example a map.

The internet is now a major resource, offering a wide variety of maps and websites which provide them for you. You are then able to print out a map and take it with you. These include:

- Multimap - http://www.multimap.com/

- Google map - http://maps.google.co.uk/maps?rls=ig&hl=en&tab=wl

- Google earth - http://earth.google.co.uk/ (you will need to download Google earth to your PC before you can use this).

Each external orientation resource, usually maps, has its positive and negative points. Although some new mobile phones have access to the internet, and therefore maps on the above websites, not everyone has one of these phones.

The A-Z is a tried, tested and successful map (a must-have for motorists).
It is portable enough to hold in your hand and I have found the maps to be the best representation of distance and proportion between buildings and places etc.

Google map is a very good resource because you can tell it where you are and where your destination is, and it can show you the route you need to find your destination – a pre-planned journey map. You can also print this map out. However, the route that this internet site will give you is only one way of getting to your destination, and does not take into account bus journeys/routes, and bus stops. There could be many reasons why the route plotted by Google maps is not the most suitable for you. You may then need to use a combination of resources.

R Routledge Taylor & Francis Group

The A-Z is also helpful when used in conjunction with timetables for public transport. Many people do not have access to or use of a car, so public transport (the bus or train), will be necessary for route finding over longer distances, for example, visiting a relative or friend who lives a distance away. You will be using bus timetables in 'Planning a night's entertainment' (Chapter 5).

It may often be necessary to use more than one route orientation resource. An example could be when visiting a friend who lives in a different part of town from you. Bus timetables are available at city travel shops, libraries or any tourist stores. These timetables will at least give you a list of the places where the bus stops, usually the name of the street. Your friend can then give you the name of the street they live in. If you know the name, you can get off the bus in the area where your friend lives, and it is then possible to work out directions using an A-Z map of that area.

Reading the A-Z involves using coordinates. Before the main route orientation activities, a coordinates training exercise is provided, to show you how to read and use coordinates in the A-Z effectively.

To plan a route on the A-Z, use a pencil to mark the direction you will walk to get there. This will involve drawing a line along the streets that you will be walking through. A sheet provided on page 111 can be photocopied for use when planning a route in this way. Look carefully in the A-Z at the streets that you walk along to get to your destination. Write the street names down on the planner sheet in the order you will come to them, to check that you are going the correct way. If you see different street names on the walk to your destination, you may be going in the wrong direction.

As mentioned, external orientation aids all have their good and bad points: for example, internet maps tend to show a particular route which may be the quickest, but not necessarily the safest. Even though internet maps are updated with some regularity, roads close and open, and often parks and even railway tracks can be in the path of your destination; and some maps are not comprehensive enough to show details which may turn out to be obstructive. Due to these potentially unforeseen dangers, it is advisable to carry a map of the area in case you are unable to use the route you originally planned to take. It is best to be prepared, to keep safe. However, roads closing and opening is a reasonably rare occurrence.

Routledge
Taylor & Francis Group

Using the A-Z

The A-Z is intended for motorists because it shows the nation's road systems. The A-Z also includes trains, street names and significant buildings, such as hospitals.

As a general rule I have found this resource to be the most reliable. However, as it is printed in book form it cannot be updated as easily as the internet map websites.

Training exercise

Before you begin the A-Z activities, a simple training exercise to demonstrate how to use this orientation resource follows.

To plan a route using the A-Z, you must firstly locate where you are starting your journey. To find an individual place, you must know the street or area name. The names of almost all streets are listed at the back of the A-Z relevant to your area. A photographic example is displayed below.

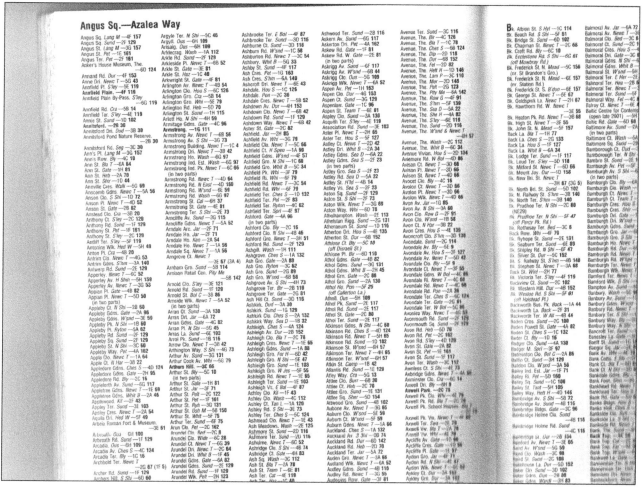

A-Z index containing all street names

When you find the place from where you are starting your journey, for example your home, it will look like this:

Mill Hill Rd. NE5: W Dent 5F **61**

The beginning of the address is the street name. The postcode for the area (NE5) follows. The postcode to an individual property, such as your home, is longer. The abbreviated area, in this case 'W Dent' (West Denton), is then given. The 5F number and letter concerns the coordinates for that part of the A-Z map. Finally there is a number in bold (61). This is the page in the A-Z where you will find the correct coordinates and location for the building or street that you are looking for.

Routledge
Taylor & Francis Group

Using coordinates

Maps in the A-Z are displayed in grids, as shown in the diagram below:

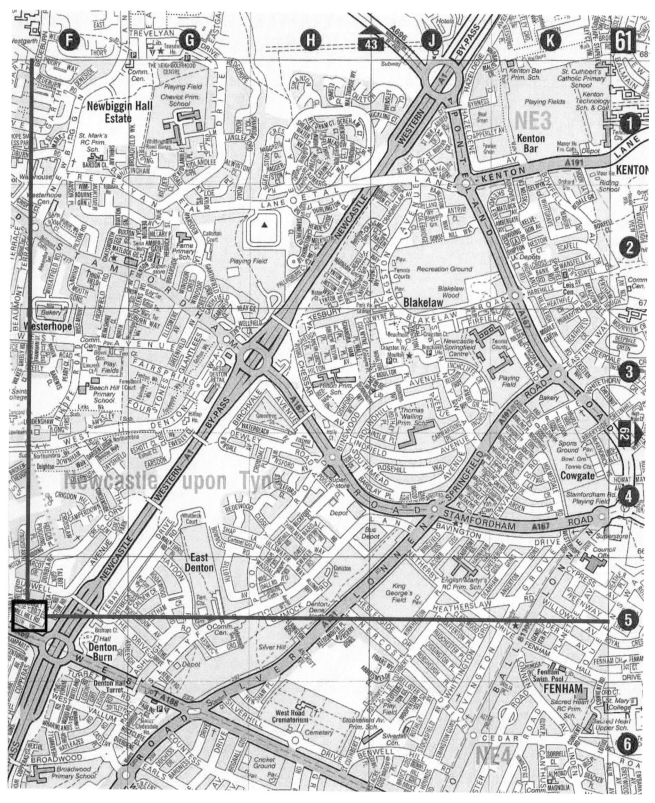

In this A-Z map example, the actual street is highlighted in the smallest black square. Coordinates only ever pinpoint a particular square of the map. The actual location that you are looking for is somewhere within that square.

In the top right hand corner is the page number 61. This is the page in the map where your destination is located. Along the side of the map are numbers and along the top are letters. The coordinate number given in the index example is 5F.

Locate number 5 in the numbers down the side of the page. Follow this number in the line of squares along the grid on the map to the left or right. The example features a red line to highlight this process.

Locate the letter along the top of the page, in this case letter F. Follow the grid down. Again, a red line is present to demonstrate this.

Eventually the lines you have made will cross each other, as in the map on the previous page. The address or place that you are searching for will be within the square where the lines have crossed.

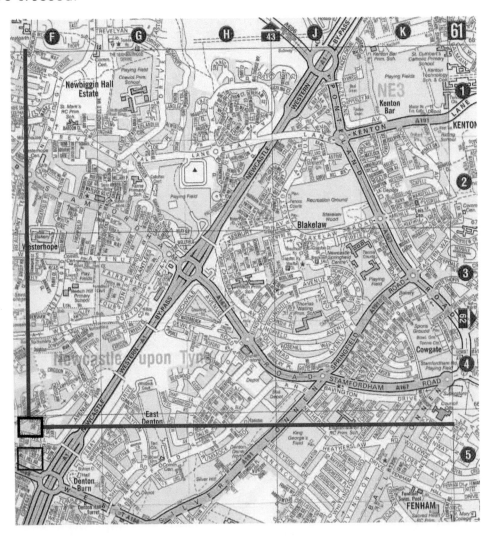

Routledge
Taylor & Francis Group

A-Z activities

Practice activity

Route orientation exercise

In the box on page 52, write down the streets and directions needed to walk from Melbourne Street, Newcastle upon Tyne to the Baltic Centre, Gateshead.

Your description should include street names and directions, left, right etc.

Put yourself in the walker's mind. An example could be, 'turn left at the end of Neville Street, then walk forward until the road ends.'

If possible, you could draw a small map using your own instructions. See how it matches up to the A-Z, or Google map / Google earth.

Ɍ Routledge
Taylor & Francis Group

Route orientation exercise

Write down the streets that you would walk along to get to The Baltic Centre, Gateshead, from Melbourne Street, Newcastle upon Tyne.

1 _____

2 _____

3 _____

4 _____

5 _____

6 _____

7 _____

8 _____

9 _____

10 _____

11 _____

12 _____

13 _____

14 _____

15 _____

16 _____

17 _____

18 _____

A-Z Activity 1

Plan a walk to St James Park football ground from Melbourne Street.

Fill in the worksheet on the next page, writing down the street names that you will walk along on the journey, in the spaces provided.

Write down the streets in the order that you come to them.

For example, on the first line at the top of the page you would write down the name of the first street you walk along, the next line will be the second street and so on. The final line will be the destination – in this case, St James Park.

A-Z Activity 1

Write down the streets you would walk along to get to St James Park from Melbourne Street.

1 _____

2 _____

3 _____

4 _____

5 _____

6 _____

7 _____

8 _____

9 _____

10 _____

11 _____

12 _____

13 _____

14 _____

15 _____

16 _____

17 _____

18 _____

Routledge Taylor & Francis Group

A-Z Activity 2

Today, you decide to go to Newcastle Arena to buy tickets to a concert.

Use the A-Z to plan your journey. Write down the names of all the streets that you will need to travel along to get to the Arena from Melbourne Street.

Use the A-Z only. Look for the safest route. The shortest distance in a city is not always the quickest or easiest! Minimise the amount of roads that you must cross on your journey to the Arena.

A-Z Activity 2

Write down the streets that you would walk along to get to Newcastle Arena from Melbourne Street.

1 _____

2 _____

3 _____

4 _____

5 _____

6 _____

7 _____

8 _____

9 _____

10 _____

11 _____

12 _____

13 _____

14 _____

15 _____

16 _____

17 _____

18 _____

Shopping centre activities

The second group of tasks in the route orientation activities are intended to give you practice at pre-trip planning. The tasks involve 'shopping trips' (4 lists). The challenge is to make the shopping trip as easily and in the shortest amount of time as possible. The map you will work from is of a large shopping centre. You will attempt to plan a route by giving the order in which you would visit places to complete the tasks.

The task initially sounds simple. However, unplanned it is very easy to go to the stores to collect the items on your list and end up passing stores that you may need to go back to later ('doubling back'). This will result in the shopping trip taking much longer than it needs to. It will also result in you walking a lot further than you need to.

Working from your shopping centre map, you must plan a shopping trip based on a shopping list that you will be given. There are four lists, each one more complex than the last. You will plan the trip, using the quickest route possible, ensuring that you will not have to pass the same store twice – which would take longer and be more tiring due to the extra walking.

Maps of the shopping centre and the store keys for both floors are presented on the next four pages. There are maps for the upper and lower floors, as you will need both to complete some shopping lists in the shortest possible time.

Routledge
Taylor & Francis Group

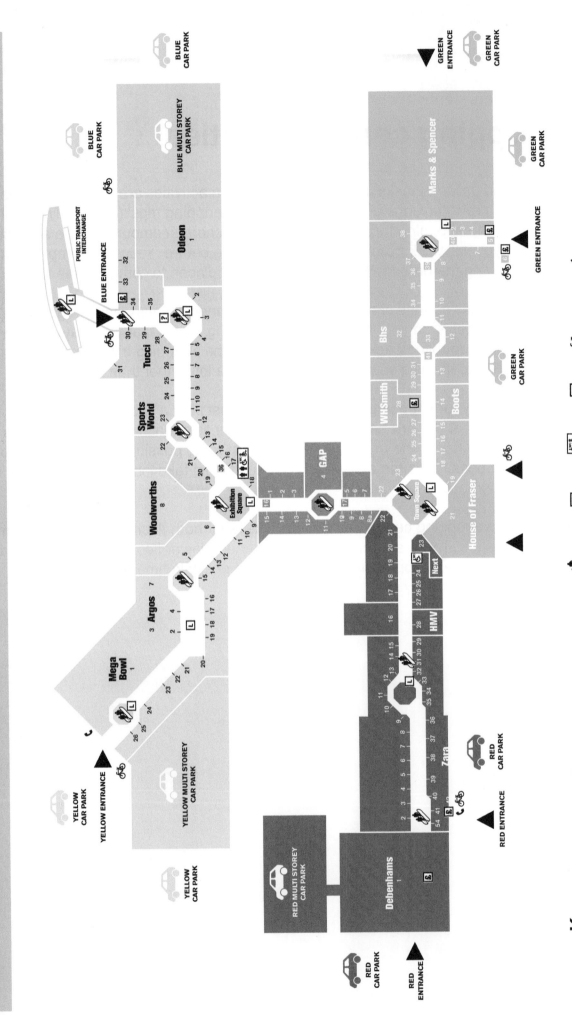

Lower Mall

MetroCentre is on 2 levels. This is the Lower Mall.

Routledge
Taylor & Francis Group

Lower Mall Category Guide

BOOKS · CARDS NEWS · STATIONERY
- Book Publishers ▲ 27
- Choices Newsagent ▲ 2
- Clinton Cards ▲ 7
- Waterstones ▲ 13
- WH Smith ▲ 28

CONFECTIONERY
- Hotel Chocolat ▲ 36
- Millies Cookies ▲ 25
- Millies Cookies ▲ 16
- Mövenpick ▲ 17
- Mövenpick ▲ 36
- Sweet Treats ▲ 26
- Sweets Galore ▲ 5
- Thorntons ▲ 17
- Walls ▲ 34

CUSTOMER SERVICES
- Alliance & Leicester £ ▲ 1
- Barclays £ ▲ 6
- Boots Pharmacy ▲ 14
- Customer Services
- HSBC £ ▲ 6
- Lloyds £ ▲ 42
- Natwest Bank (+£) ▲ 4
- Natwest £ ▲ 6
- Northern Rock £ ▲ 33
- Northern Rock £ ▲ 42
- RAC ▲ 41

DEPARTMENT & VARIETY STORES
- Argos Extra ▲ 3
- Bhs ▲ 32
- Boots ▲ 14
- Debenhams ▲ 1
- Disney Store ▲ 5
- House of Fraser ▲ 21
- Marks & Spencer ▲ 1
- Next ▲ 23
- Primark ▲ 16
- Superdrug ▲ 27
- Woolworths ▲ 8

ELECTRICAL GOODS & MUSIC COMMUNICATION – IT
- 3 Store ▲ 19
- BT ▲ 40
- Carphone Warehouse ▲ 9
- Carphone Warehouse ▲ 29
- Currys Digital ▲ 38
- Game ▲ 20
- Gamestation ▲ 25
- HMV ▲ 28
- LE Concepts ▲ 21
- O2 ▲ 23
- Orange ▲ 40
- Phones 4 U ▲ 6
- Phones 4 U ▲ 17
- Virgin ▲ 34
- Virgin Mobile ▲ 11
- Vodafone ▲ 8
- Williams Music ▲ 20

ENTERTAINMENT & LEISURE
- Disney Store ▲ 5
- Megabowl ▲ 1
- Odeon Cinemas ▲ 1
- Quasar ▲ 7
- William Hill ▲ 32

FASHION & ACCESSORIES

Childrens
- Base ▲ 9
- French Connection ▲ 4
- Gap kids/Baby Gap ▲ 4
- Monsoon ▲ 37
- Mothercare ▲ 1
- USC ▲ 5

Ladies
- Ann Harvey ▲ 12
- Bay Trading ▲ 8
- Bay Trading ▲ 25
- Coast ▲ 33
- Fashion Express ▲ 19
- Internacionale ▲ 7
- Jane Norman ▲ 20
- Karen Millen ▲ 2
- Kookai (within House of Fraser) ▲ 21
- La Senza Lingerie ▲ 15
- Mango ▲ 41
- Monsoon ▲ 37
- Principles ▲ 11
- Quiz ▲ 24
- Rebel Rebel ▲ 11
- Top Shop ▲ 12
- Zara ▲ 38

Mens
- Base ▲ 9
- Burton ▲ 9
- Cecil Gee ▲ 35
- Envy ▲ 11
- Suits You ▲ 3
- The Officer's Club ▲ 9
- Youngs Hire ▲ 3

Mixed
- French Connection ▲ 4
- Gap ▲ 4
- H & M ▲ 6
- Kickers ▲ 31
- Lacoste ▲ 15
- Next ▲ 23
- Primark ▲ 16
- Republic ▲ 7
- River Island ▲ 37
- Scotts ▲ 14
- Tucci Man & Woman ▲ 26
- USC ▲ 5
- Zara ▲ 38

Specialist & Accessories
- Accessorize ▲ 16
- Ann Summers ▲ 27
- Claire's Accessories ▲ 18
- Claire's Accessories ▲ 18
- Scotts ▲ 14
- Sunglass Hut ▲ 39
- Tie Rack ▲ 8
- Watch Station ▲ 39

FOOD
- Greggs ▲ 29
- Holland & Barratt ▲ 14
- Marks & Spencer ▲ 1

HAIR & BEAUTY
- Brokyn Barbering Company ▲ 19
- Trade Secret ▲ 12

JEWELLERY
- Beaverbrooks ▲ 22
- Earnest Jones ▲ 18
- Fraser Hart ▲ 13
- Goldsmiths ▲ 3
- Goldsmiths ▲ 24
- H Samuel ▲ 26
- Market Cross ▲ 2
- Mayfair ▲ 13
- Swarovski ▲ 30
- Warren James ▲ 30

OPTICIANS
- Boots ▲ 14
- Super Optical ▲ 7

RESTAURANTS · CAFES · BARS
- Bhs ▲ 32
- Burger King ▲ 21
- Café Gio ▲ 33
- Chiquito ▲ 30
- Debenhams ▲ 15
- Est ▲ 23
- Marks & Spencer ▲ 16
- McDonalds ▲ 7
- McDonalds ▲ 37
- McDonalds ▲ 14
- Milligans ▲ 26
- Muffin Break ▲ 5
- Nandos ▲ 38
- Pizza Hut ▲ 16
- Queen Vic ▲ 27
- Quiznos ▲ 18
- Ricardo's ▲ 18
- Rollover ▲ 14
- Zee Zee Fresh Juices & Smoothies ▲ 5

SHOES
- Barratts ▲ 22
- Clarks ▲ 17
- Dolcis ▲ 8a
- Dune ▲ 32
- Faith ▲ 35
- Garage Shoes ▲ 13
- Jones Bootmaker ▲ 36
- Liberta ▲ 21
- Schuh ▲ 39

SPECIALIST SHOPS
- Au Naturale ▲ 5
- Build a Bear ▲ 14
- Body Shop ▲ 19
- Body Shop ▲ 13
- Carsmart ▲ 23
- Collectables ▲ 15
- Florida Print ▲ 17
- Garden Mews ▲ 18
- Herbal Inn ▲ 12
- Herbal Inn ▲ 24
- Herbs & Acupuncture ▲ 15
- Hoover Service ▲ 22
- Madhouse ▲ 2
- Parker Tools ▲ 24
- Poundworld ▲ 22
- Swarovski ▲ 30
- Timpson ▲ 3
- Timpson ▲ 26
- Watch Repair Centre ▲ 16

SPORTS & OUTDOORS
- First Sport ▲ 10
- JD Sports ▲ 15
- Newcastle United FC ▲ 10
- Newcastle Wrestling Store ▲ 4
- Scotts ▲ 14
- Sports World ▲ 23

TOYS · GAMES · HOBBIES
- Disney Store ▲ 5

TRAVEL AGENTS
- Going Places ▲ 8

Finding your way around

MetroCentre is divided into colours malls, Red, Blue, Green and Yellow, co-ordinating with the nearest free car park, and two floors – upper mall and lower mall. They are linked by Central mall which is coloured grey on the map.

If you get lost or separated we suggest you meet by the Customer Services Desk, ground floor.

Green Mall next to Marks and Spencer. We can only make special announcements to lost children and serious emergencies.

▲ = Lower Mall
▲ = Central Mall
£ = Cash Machines

Routledge
Taylor & Francis Group

Upper Mall

MetroCentre is on 2 levels. This is the Upper Mall.

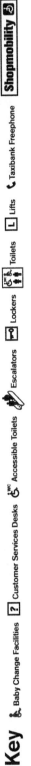

ACCESS TO COACH PARK
AND RAILWAY STATION

PUBLIC TRANSPORT
INTERCHANGE

BLUE ENTRANCE

BLUE MULTI STOREY
CAR PARK

The Village

The Forum

Collectables

Costa

Vision Express

Sports World

Woolworths

Evans

MetroFood Court
temporarily closed

The New Metroland

YELLOW ENTRANCE

YELLOW MULTI STOREY
CAR PARK

THE STUDIO

The Studio

WHSmith

House of Fraser

New Look

ScS

HMV

Next

Zara

Debenhams

RED MULTI STOREY
CAR PARK

RED ENTRANCE

Key

Baby Change Facilities
Customer Services Desks
Accessible Toilets
Escalators
Lockers
Toilets
Lifts
Taxibank Freephone
Shopmobility

Routledge
Taylor & Francis Group

Upper Mall Category Guide

Remember, more shops, more time to shop. MetroCentre Opening Hours:

BOOKS • CARDS / NEWS • STATIONERY
- Best Wishes △ 15
- Birthdays △ 24
- The Works △ 23
- Topics △ 34
- Waterstones △ 17
- WH Smith △ 20
- WH Smith △ 30

CONFECTIONERY
- Marcantonios △ 15
- Sweet Factory △ 16
- Walls - Swirl It △ 8

CUSTOMER SERVICES
- Abbey (+£) ▲ 1
- Barclays £ ▲ 44
- Chapel † △ V16
- Dentist △ 27
- Halifax PLC (+£) ▲ 41
- HSBC £ △ 12
- Lloyds £ ▲ 47
- New Stitch △ F3
- Northern Rock £ △ 31
- Northumbria Police △ 28
- Post Office ▲ 34
- Quickstitch △ 9
- Shopmobility △ 33
- Travel Shop △ 32

DEPARTMENT & VARIETY STORES
- Boots ▲ 10
- Debenhams ▲ 1
- House of Fraser △ 15
- Next ▲ 38
- Woolworths △ 6

ELECTRICAL GOODS & MUSIC COMMUNICATION – IT
- 3 Store △ 18
- Carphone Warehouse ▲ 39
- Computer Solutionz △ F13
- Future Fone Citi △ F8
- Game ▲ 48
- HMV ▲ 40
- Linetone Audio △ 26
- Maughan Micro ▲ 45
- Mobile Phone Repair Shop △ 14
- O2 ▲ 32
- Orange △ 12
- Sony Centre ▲ 31
- T Mobile △ 16
- T Mobile Specialists/Fone House △ 11
- Vodafone

ENTERTAINMENT & LEISURE
- Mr B's Amusements △ 17
- The New MetroLand △ 1

FASHION & ACCESSORIES

Childrens
- Monsoon △ 33
- Mothercare △ 1
- Peek A Boo △ 15
- Pumkin Patch ▲ 4
- Zara ▲ 51

Ladies
- Bershka ▲ 52
- CC Fashions △ V17
- Dorothy Perkins ▲ 4
- Elvi △ 23
- Evans △ 5
- EWM (Edinburgh Woollen Mill) △ 16
- Laura Ashley △ 6
- Miss Selfridge △ 7
- Mk △ 20
- Monsoon △ 33
- New Image △ F4
- Oasis △ 16
- Paris △ 31
- Wallis △ 5
- Warehouse ▲ 11

Mens
- Aston △ 4
- EWM (Edinburgh Woollen Mill) △ 16
- GW △ 7
- Jack & Jones ▲ 46
- Leftfield △ 13
- Modo & Pelle △ 28
- The Officer's Club △ 7
- Top Man △ 7
- Zara ▲ 51

Mixed
- Doc Black △ X
- G-Star Raw △ X
- H&M ▲ X
- NewLook ▲ X
- Next ▲ X
- Original Shoe Co. △ X
- River Island ▲ 50
- Zara ▲ 51

Specialist & Accessories
- Completely Bonkers △ V14
- Demure Leather △ 8
- Milano ▲ F1
- Petit Diable ▲ F5
- Skate Shack ▲ F9
- Tights Tights Tights △ 29
- Triple S ▲ 30
- Triple S △ 14
- Xtras ▲ F10

FOOD
- Greggs △ 29
- Old Fizzywigs △ V3

HAIR & BEAUTY
- Bodycare ▲ 21
- Hair Express ▲ 14
- Hot Hair - Fashion wigs and hairpieces △ V10
- Regis Hair & Beauty △ 8
- Sherlocks Hairdressing ▲ F12
- Supercuts △ 36
- The Barber Shop △ V15
- The Original Barber Shop △ 11
- The Perfume Shop ▲ 5
- The Perfume Shop △ 22
- Toni & Guy △ 8

JEWELLERY
- Christopher James ▲ 22
- David Summerfield △ 27
- Goldsmiths △ 17
- HPJ The Jeweller ▲ 21
- Mulroy Antiques △ V6
- Muse △ 6

OPTICIANS
- Dollond & Aitchison △ 15
- Optical Express △ 13
- Vision Express ▲ 25

RESTAURANTS • CAFES • BARS
- Big Lukes △ 1
- Big Lukes △ S7
- Buffet King @ Metro ▲ 25
- Burger King △ 18
- Café Nova △ 26
- Café Rouge ▲ 14
- Cafe Studio △ S9
- Cookery Nook △ 35
- Costa Coffee △ F11
- Costa Coffee (within WH Smith) △ 20a
- Debenhams ▲ 1
- El Molino △ S5
- El Porko ▲ S1
- House of Fraser △ 15
- KFC △ 2
- Madisons ▲ 36
- Madisons ▲ 37
- Massarella △ 25
- Massarella ▲ 30
- McDonalds △ 2
- Metro Food Court Temporarily Closed
- Mocha △ 2
- Petit Delice △ 12
- Ping On II △ S3
- Romanos △ S2
- Starbucks △ S8
- Spice Bollywood △ 7
- Sweet Sensations ▲ S4
- Sweet Sensations in The Village △ V1
- Wetherspoons △ V21
- Wetherspoons △ 26

SHOES
- DocBlacl △ V9
- Durham Shoe Box ▲ V2
- Priceless Shoes △ 9
- Russell & Bromley △ 19
- Shoe Zone ▲ 12
- Skate Shack ▲ F9

SPECIALIST SHOPS
- Appletree Bonsai △ V19
- Baileys Blinds △ V4
- Collectables ▲ 32
- Collectables Oven to Table △ 3
- Compliments △ F14
- Computer Solutionz ▲ F13
- Confetti Bridal △ F2
- Forget Flowers △ 10
- Genghis International △ F7
- Hot Hair - Fashion wigs and hairpieces △ V10
- Isis Aromatherapy ▲ V5
- Isis - Mind, Body, Spirit △ V12
- Jessops △ 34
- JustPink △ 9
- La Galleria D'Art △ 13
- Lush △ 35
- Magic Box ▲ 10
- Photography for Little People △ 4
- Poundland ▲ 5
- Rosebys △ V8
- Scotch Corner △ 6
- SCS Furnishings ▲ V11
- Specialist Mirror Shop ▲ V18
- streetcred.biz △ V20
- The Elizabethan ▲ V11
- The Lindisfarne Room incorporating The Specialist Mirror Shop
- The Paper Mill Shop ▲ 4
- The Pier ▲ 54
- The Professional Cookware Company △ 53
- The Whisky Shop △ 33
- Transform your images △ 13

SPORTS & OUTDOORS
- Blacks △ 24
- Dancesport & Equestrian △ 9
- EWM (The Golf Company) △ 16
- F1 Racing Gear △ 11
- JD Sports ▲ 10
- Millets △ 3
- Sports World △ 19

TOYS • GAMES • HOBBIES
- Early Learning Centre ▲ 2
- Game ▲ 48
- Games Workshop △ 29
- Grainger Games △ V7
- Mind Games ▲ F6
- Model Zone ▲ 42

TRAVEL AGENTS
- Thomas Cook ▲ 14
- Thomas Cook ▲ 43
- Thomson △ 5

Finding your way around

MetroCentre is divided into colours malls, Red, Blue, Green and Yellow, co-ordinating with the nearest free car park, and two floors - upper mall and lower mall. They are linked by Central mall which is coloured grey on the map.

If you get lost or separated we suggest you meet by the Customer Services Desk, ground floor, Green Mall next to Marks and Spencer. We can only make special announcements for lost children and serious emergencies.

▲ ▲ ▲ Upper Mall
△ △ △ Central Mall
£ = Cash Machines

Routledge
Taylor & Francis Group

Shopping list A

In the box that follows, write down the order in which you would visit the places to complete your shopping in the shortest time possible.

Enter the MetroCentre at the blue quadrant, lower floor.

1 Greggs for two cheese pasties.

2 Post Office to post a parcel.

3 Sports World, to buy a football.

4 Watch a magic show in the town square.

5 Gap to buy a shirt.

Exit the MetroCentre at the blue quadrant, lower floor.

Routledge Taylor & Francis Group

Shopping list A cont'd

Write down the order in which you would visit the places on your list to complete your shopping in the shortest time possible.

Enter the MetroCentre at the blue quadrant, lower floor.

1

2

3

4

5

Exit the MetroCentre at the blue quadrant, lower floor.

Shopping list B

Enter the MetroCentre at the red quadrant, lower floor.

1 Withdraw money from a cash machine.

2 Buy a music CD from HMV.

3 Buy socks at Primark.

4 Buy a birthday card from Clinton Cards.

5 Have a key cut at Timpson.

6 Phone a taxi to take you home.

Exit the MetroCentre at the red quadrant, lower floor.

Routledge
Taylor & Francis Group

Shopping list B cont'd

Write down the order in which you would visit the stores on your list to complete your shopping in the shortest possible time.

Enter the MetroCentre at the red quadrant, lower floor.

1

2

3

4

5

Exit the MetroCentre at the red quadrant, lower floor.

Shopping list C

Begin at the bus and train concourse at the blue quadrant.

1 Bank, to take some cash out of your Abbey savings account.

2 Deodorant.

3 A copy of *Empire* magazine.

4 A quick coffee, to 'keep you going'.

5 Baby clothes for a relative's child.

6 Pair of jeans.

7 Two t-shirts.

8 Some basic groceries / food shopping.

9 *I Am Legend* on DVD.

10 Duffy's album on CD.

11 Book of stamps.

12 A nice piece of jewellery for an elderly lady's birthday.

Routledge
Taylor & Francis Group

Shopping list C cont'd

First make a list of the stores you will visit to complete your shopping, and then write down the order in which you would visit the stores on your list to complete your shopping in the shortest time possible.

Stores on two levels have in-store stairs, so you can use these.

Enter the MetroCentre at the blue quadrant, lower floor.

1 _____

2 _____

3 _____

4 _____

5 _____

6 _____

7 _____

8 _____

9 _____

10 _____

11 _____

12 _____

Exit the MetroCentre at the blue quadrant, upper floor.

Shopping list D

Enter the MetroCentre at the blue quadrant, lower floor.

1 Upgrade O2 mobile phone.

2 Tie Rack for red silk tie.

3 Parker Tools for hammer and nails.

4 Disney Store for Mickey Mouse toy.

5 Quickstitch for trouser alterations.

6 Thorntons for special chocolates.

7 Buffet King for lunch.

8 The Paper Mill Shop for red, shiny paper.

9 Early Learning Centre for child's game.

10 Collectables for china pony.

11 EWM to buy a woollen scarf.

12 Poundland for six items at £1 each.

13 Model Zone for scale model of space shuttle.

14 Professional Cookware Company for a set of pans.

Exit the MetroCentre at the blue quadrant, lower floor.

Routledge
Taylor & Francis Group

Shopping list D cont'd

Write down the order in which you would visit the stores on your list to complete your shopping in the shortest time possible.

Enter the MetroCentre at the blue quadrant, lower floor.

1 _____

2 _____

3 _____

4 _____

5 _____

6 _____

7 _____

8 _____

9 _____

10 _____

11 _____

12 _____

13 _____

14 _____

Exit the MetroCentre at the blue quadrant, upper floor.

Routledge
Taylor & Francis Group

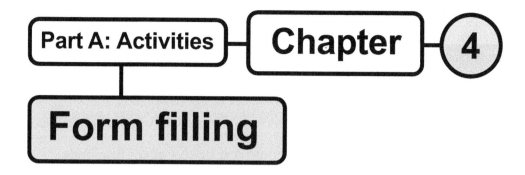

Part A: Activities — Chapter — 4

Form filling

Filling in forms is not exactly fun, but it is a skill that you will probably use many times in your life. Forms generally have the purpose of enabling you to obtain something you want by disclosing information about yourself.

Form examples:

- Job applications
- Opening a bank account
- Obtaining a passport or bus pass
- Joining a club or organisation
- Applications for store discount cards.

As a general rule, forms consist of a series of boxes or lines following requests for information, eg 'Name', and you will write your name in the box or on the lines provided. Each line or box will require a different answer about a piece of personal information about yourself. Opposite is what a typical form looks like.

Many forms are very strict in the way they want you to present the information, because completed forms are often scanned into a computer, and some computers will only recognise black ink, so the letters or words presented must be clear.

A typical form

Routledge
Taylor & Francis Group

Living with an Acquired Brain Injury

A job application form may ask for your details to be presented in blue ink, and if you use another colour, it may show to a potential future employer that you cannot read instructions. However, as a general rule, black ink is asked for most often. This may be for many reasons. It is important to follow instructions as closely as possible. If you do not, it may take your form longer to process or cause difficulty at some stage in the form's processing.

Forms will require you to put your personal information into the boxes or on the lines provided. Typically, a form will first ask for your name, date of birth and age, address, and job title. It is not possible to supply a complete list of the information required in all cases, as all forms differ. Therefore, before completing a form, it is a good idea to have a quick look at the information needed, and put all the required documentation together. That way it is easier to complete the form in one sitting, as you will have all the necessary information to hand.

Most forms include some basic instructions at the beginning, eg 'use a black pen', 'all writing in block capitals' and so on. The more complicated and lengthy forms will have considerably more instructions. Some forms can be so complicated that they will have a page of instructions before the form begins. Some forms are very long, for example the passport application form, which is so long in fact that instead of an instruction page on the form, it comes with a full instruction booklet, which is almost as long as the form itself.

Some forms you will be required to complete may ask for information a little more complex than just single word or number answers. In this case, you will be given a larger box or series of lines to fill in with the more complicated and in-depth personal information. Block capitals are usually required to fill in this section and indeed are recommended, as lower case letters in handwriting can be harder to read and may slow the processing of your application form.

Sometimes a large box, or many lines for complex information, may still not be enough space for the information the form requires. Due to the methods used to scan or photocopy the forms, any information written out of the box or lines may be chopped off. The usual course of action here, and one which is most often requested in the instructions for completing the form, is to add any extra information on a separate piece of paper, and attach it to the form. A paperclip or stapler may be used to do this and it will be necessary to write in the box, 'See attached sheet for further information'. Always read and follow form instructions as closely as possible.

Time to practise filling in some forms…

 Routledge Taylor & Francis Group

Bank account application form activity

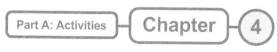

Delta Bank

INSTANT SAVER ACCOUNT - APPLICATION FORM

Fill in form using BLOCK CAPITALS and black ink.   ✔ Tick any boxes which apply

First Applicant	Second Applicant
Title: Mr ☐ Mrs ☐ Ms ☐ Other ☐	Title: Mr ☐ Mrs ☐ Ms ☐ Other ☐
Surname:	Surname:
Forenames:	Forenames:
Address:	Address:
Postcode:	Postcode:
Time at current address: years ☐ months ☐	Time at current address: years ☐ months ☐
Date of birth: ___ / ___ / ___ dd/mm/yy	Date of birth: ___ / ___ / ___ dd/mm/yy
Town of birth:	Town of birth:
Country of birth:	Country of birth:
Home no. :	Home no. :
Mobile/Other:	Mobile/Other:
Email:	Email:
Marital status:	Marital status:
Mother's maiden name:	Mother's maiden name:
At the above address are you:	At the above address are you:
Owner occupier ☐ Living with parents ☐	Owner occupier ☐ Living with parents ☐
Tenant ☐ Other ☐	Tenant ☐ Other ☐
If 'owner occupier', Approximate market value of your home: £	If 'owner occupier', Approximate market value of your home: £
Mortgage outstanding: £	Mortgage outstanding: £

Delta Bank

Ⓡ Routledge
Taylor & Francis Group

Living with an Acquired Brain Injury

Store loyalty card application form activity

Sign Up Today
COMPLETE IN BLOCK CAPITALS
USING A BLACK PEN

RONTO

RONTO DISCOUNT AND POINTS CARD

RONTO REWARDS NO.	RONTO **STORE OF CARD APPLICATION:**
26.6.81.29	MERSON BRANCH, VIVELCHESTER

Email address

Title (Mr, Mrs, Miss, Ms)

First name:

Surname:

Company name:

Address:

Postcode:

Phone number:

RONTO

Routledge Taylor & Francis Group

Concessionary bus pass activity

BUS PASS

Name

Is this your first concessionary bus pass?

Is this a replacement pass submission request?

Date of birth [D.O.B.]

Address

Postcode

Eligibility (disabled, senior citizen, etc)

Telephone number

First line of previous address (if applicable)

HAVE YOU PROVIDED:	TICK
Bill addressed to you (Phone bill including mobile or utility bills, are suitable for this) (Photocopies of these official documents are permitted)	
Council tax bill (as secondary evidence of residence) (Photocopies of this bill are permitted)	

Routledge
Taylor & Francis Group

Living with an Acquired Brain Injury

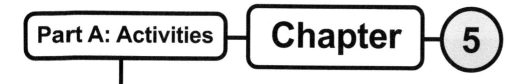

Planning a night's entertainment

This chapter does not involve sitting in front of the TV, but planning a night out of the house. Even if this is not the way you would usually spend an evening, the activities will help to build your organisational skills, and include:

- Timing

- Planning

- Basic research examples

- Using resources.

The first important skill you should master is understanding the 24-hour clock. This will help you to read transport, cinema, theatre and other timetables that you will probably encounter. An example of how to read and understand a 24-hour clock follows. It is recommended that you spend the first part of this section learning how to read the 24-hour clock.

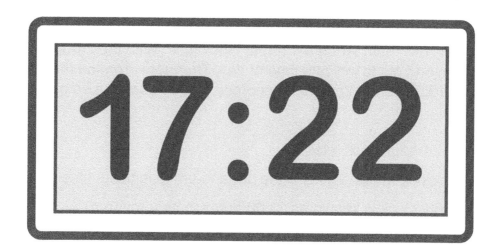

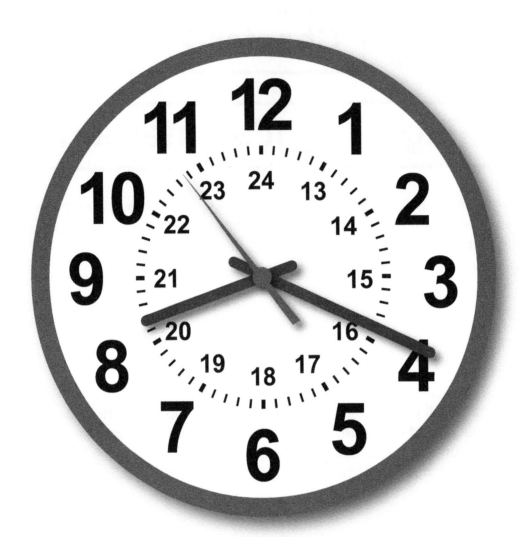

Above is a large picture of a 24-hour analogue clock. The 24-hour clock is based on each hour having its own number on a 12-hour clock face. With the 24-hour clock we do not need the am and pm to indicate time of day. Therefore, 1pm on the 24-hour clock is known as 13:00 hours, 2pm then becomes 14:00 hours and so on until 24:00 hours (midnight).

Memory jogger for 24-hour clock rules:

- With the 24-hour clock we do not need the am and pm to indicate time of day.

- 1pm on the 24-hour clock is known as 13:00 hours instead of 1pm.

- 2pm then becomes 14:00 hours and so on until 24:00 hours (midnight).

- Then at 1am the cycle begins again for another day.

 R Routledge
Taylor & Francis Group

24-hour clock activities

You will need to use this bus timetable to answer the questions in the activities that follow.

Monday to Friday													
Four Lane Ends Metro	1939	1954	2009	2004	2039	2054	2109	2124	2139	2154	2207	2221	2236
Coach Lane Campus	1941	1956	2011	2026	2041	2056	2111	2126	2141	2156	2209	2223	2238
Cochrane Park	1943	1958	2013	2028	2043	2058	2113	2128	2143	2158	2211	2225	2240
Chillingham Road Shops	1948	2003	2018	2033	2048	2103	2118	2133	2148	2203	2216	2230	2246
Sandyford	1959	2014	2029	2044	2059	2114	2129	2144	2159	2214	2227	2241	2256
Haymarket John Dobson Street	2002	2017	2032	2047	2102	2117	2135	2147	2202	2217	2230	2244	2258
Monument Pligrim Street	2004	2019	2034	2049	2104	2119	2134	2149	2204	2219	2232	2246	2300
Monument Market Street	2005	2020	2035	2050	2105	2120	2135	2150	2205	2220	2233	2247	2301
Central Station Neville Street ..	2009	2024	2039	2054	2109	2124	2139	2154	2209	2224	2237	2251	2305
Cruddas Park	2014	2029	2044	2059	2114	2129	2144	2159	2214	2229	2241	2255	2309
South Benwell	2016	2031	2046	2101	2116	2131	2146	2201	2216	2231	2243	2257	2311
Scotswood	2022	2037	2052	2107	2122	2137	2152	2207	2222	2237	2249	2303	2315
Whickham View	2024	2039	2034	2109	2124	2139	2154	2209	2224	2239	2251	2305	2317
Denton Burn	2026	2041	2056	2111	2126	2141	2156	2211	2226	2241	2253	2307	2321
Slatyford	2029	2044	2059	2114	2129	2144	2159	2214	2229	2244	2256	2310	2324

Give the answers using the 24-hour clock, and then convert them to the 12-hour clock. An example is:

Bus leaves Four Lane Ends Metro at 19:39.

What time does it arrive at Slatyford?

24-hour clock 20:29 12-hour clock 8.29pm.

Routledge
Taylor & Francis Group

24-hour clock activities

Bus leaves Coach Lane Campus at 19:56.

What time does it arrive at Cruddas Park?

24-hour clock [   ]   **12-hour clock** [   ]

Bus leaves Cochrane Park at 20:28.

What time does it arrive at Denton Burn?

24-hour clock [   ]   **12-hour clock** [   ]

Bus leaves Sandyford at 21:14.

What time does it arrive at Whickham View?

24-hour clock [   ]   **12-hour clock** [   ]

Bus leaves Chillingham Road shops at 21:33.

What time does it arrive at Scotswood?

24-hour clock [   ]   **12-hour clock** [   ]

Bus leaves Haymarket John Dobson Street at 22:02.

What time does it arrive at Slatyford?

24-hour clock [   ]   **12-hour clock** [   ]

 Routledge
Taylor & Francis Group

24-hour clock activities cont'd

What time is the last bus from Sandyford?

24-hour clock [   ]   **12-hour clock** [   ]

What time does the last bus arrive at Slatyford?

24-hour clock [   ]   **12-hour clock** [   ]

Night out entertainment planning / activity

In the following activity you will plan your night of entertainment. These example activities and elements of the night out may not be to your taste. However, using them as examples of planning and organising a night out will still allow you to develop skills that you will find beneficial. This example night out will consist of planning and organising the following:

- Mode of transport (bus or taxi)

- Cinema

- Restaurant.

If a night out depends on public transport, it will be necessary to plan to complete the various activities in a certain length of time. What time is the last bus home?

Even if a night out does not depend on public transport, it will still be necessary to plan to complete the various activities in a certain time frame because of closing times, for example:

- Will you have time for a meal?

- Will you eat before or after the film?

This activity will give you some practice at this type of planning.

The activity

- The activity for this session involves planning the night out.

- You must fill in the 'activity worksheet'. The activities and other 'night out' elements must be planned as to what happens when.

- You are required to write the times you will start and end an activity – cinema, meal and transport.

- You will need to use the three timetables you will be given: a separate timetable for the meal, cinema times and bus.

Living with an Acquired Brain Injury

R Routledge
Taylor & Francis Group

Night out entertainment activities

- Public transport into town.
- A trip to the cinema to see a film.
- A meal at 'Pizza Kitchen'.
- A bus or taxi home.

Night out planner

- Use the sheet on the next page to plan your night out.
- Start with the time that your bus leaves Chapel House.
- Do you want to eat before or after the film?
- Make sure you allow time between activities to get there.
- Can you catch the last bus home or will you need to book a taxi?
- Under the name of each part of the night (eg bus, meal), write the number of the bus or the name of the restaurant.

Activity worksheet

Bus	Start:
	Arrive:

Meal	Start:
	End:

Cinema	Start:
	End:

Transport	Start:
	Return home:

Resources

To complete this task, you will need the following resources (examples displayed):

- Bus timetable
- Cinema times
- 'Pizza Kitchen' menu.

 Routledge Taylor & Francis Group

Bus timetable

Effective From: 04 October 2009 Service

Vivelchester - Newcastle – Westerhope – Chapel House: Bus No. 35

Monday to Friday

Vivelchester	0649	0719	0749	*19	49	1719	1749	1819	1846	1946	2046	2146	2246
Newcastle Newgate Street	0651	0721	0751	*21	51	1721	1751	1821	1848	1948	2048	2148	2248
Newcastle St James	0652	0722	0752	*22	52	1722	1752	1822	1849	1949	2049	2149	2249
BBC TV Centre	0656	0726	0756	*26	56	1726	1756	1826	1853	1953	2053	2153	2253
Cowgate	0700	0730	0800	*30	00	1730	1800	1830	1857	1957	2057	2157	2257
Slatyford	0703	0733	0803	*33	03	1733	1803	1833	1900	2000	2100	2200	2300
Westerhope	0708	0738	0808	*38	08	1738	1808	1838	1905	2005	2105	2205	2305
Chapel House	0715	0745	0815	*45	15	1745	1815	1845	1912	2012	2112	2212	2312

Saturday

Vivelchester	0629	0819	0849	*19	49	1719	1749	1819	1846	1946	2046	2146	2246
Newcastle Newgate Street	0631	0821	0851	*21	51	1721	1751	1821	1848	1948	2048	2148	2248
Newcastle St James	0632	0822	0852	*22	52	1722	1752	1822	1849	1949	2049	2149	2249
BBC TV Centre	0636	0826	0856	*26	56	1726	1756	1826	1853	1953	2053	2153	2253
Cowgate	0640	0830	0900	*30	00	1730	1800	1830	1857	1957	2057	2157	2257
Slatyford	0643	0833	0903	*33	03	1733	1803	1833	1900	2000	2100	2200	2300
Westerhope	0648	0838	0908	*38	08	1738	1808	1838	1905	2005	2105	2205	2305
Chapel House	0655	0845	0915	*45	15	1745	1815	1845	1912	2012	2112	2212	2312

Sunday

Vivelchester		0946	*46	2246
Newcastle Newgate Street	0736	0806	0948	*48	2248
Newcastle St James	0737	0807	0949	*49	2249
BBC TV Centre	0741	0811	0953	*53	2253
Cowgate	0745	0815	0957	*57	2257
Slatyford	0748	0818	1000	*00	2300
Westerhope	0753	0823	1005	*05	2305
Chapel House	0759	0829	1012	*12	2312

Timetable key:
* : Then at these minutes past each hour.........until:

Routledge
Taylor & Francis Group

Bus timetable

Effective From: 04 October 2009 Service

Chapel House – Westerhope – Newcastle – Vivelchester: Bus No. 35

Monday to Friday

Chapel House	0652	0718	0748	*18	48	1718	1748	1818	1913	2013	2113	2213	2312
Westerhope	0659	0725	0755	*25	55	1725	1755	1825	1920	2020	2120	2220	2318
Slatyford	0704	0730	0800	*30	00	1730	1800	1830	1925	2025	2125	2225	2322
Cowgate	0707	0733	0803	*33	03	1733	1803	1833	1928	2028	2128	2228	–
BBC TV Centre	0711	0737	0807	*37	07	1737	1807	1837	1932	2032	2132	2232	–
Central Station Westgate Road	0717	0743	0813	*43	13	1743	1813	1843	1938	2038	2138	2238	–
Newcastle Newgate Street	0718	0744	0814	*44	14	1744	1814	1844	1939	2039	2139	2239	–
Vivelchester	0721	0751	0821	*51	21	1751	1821	1848	1948	2048	2148	2248	–

Saturday

Chapel House	0601	0701	0731	0748	0818	0848	*18	48	1718	1748	1818	1913	2013	2113	2213	2312
Westerhope	0607	0707	0737	0755	0825	0855	*25	55	1725	1755	1825	1920	2020	2120	2220	2318
Slatyford	0612	0712	0742	0800	0830	0900	*30	00	1730	1800	1830	1925	2025	2125	2225	2322
Cowgate	0615	0715	0745	0803	0833	0903	*33	03	1733	1803	1833	1928	2028	2128	2228	–
BBC TV Centre	0619	0719	0749	0807	0837	0907	*37	07	1737	1807	1837	1932	2032	2132	2232	–
Newcastle St James	0723	–	–	–	–	–	–	–	–	–	–	–	–	–	–	–
Newcastle Monument	0724	–	–	–	–	–	–	–	–	–	–	–	–	–	–	–
Central Station Westgate Road	0625	–	–	0755	0813	0843	0913	*43	13	1743	1813	1843	1938	2038	2138	2238
Newcastle Newgate Street	0626	–	–	0756	0814	0844	0914	*44	14	1744	1814	1844	1939	2039	2139	2239
Vivelchester	0631	–	–	0801	0821	0851	0921	*51	21	1751	1821	1848	1948	2048	2148	2248

Sunday

Chapel House	0731	0801	0831	0913	*13	2213	2312
Westerhope	0737	0807	0837	0920	*20	2220	2318
Slatyford	0742	0812	0842	0925	*25	2225	2322
Cowgate	0745	0815	0845	0928	*28	2228	
BBC TV Centre	0749	0819	0849	0932	*32	2232	
Newcastle St James	0753	0823	0853	–		–	
Newcastle Monument	0754	0824	0854	–		–	
Central Station Westgate Road				0938	*38	2238	
Newcastle Newgate Street				0939	*39	2239	
Vivelchester				0948	*48	2248	

> **Timetable key:**
> * : Then at these minutes past each hour.........until:

Cinema times

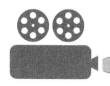

Vivel Screen Cinema: Vivelchester

Thunder
Running time: 107 mins
Friday 26/09/08
11.50   14.15   16.45   19.10   21.35

Pineapple Express
Running time: 111 mins
Friday 26/09/08
13.45   16.15   18.45   21.15

Mamma Mia!
Running time: 109 mins
Friday 26/09/08
11.50   14.15   16.45   19.10   21.35

Mamma Mia! (Sing-a-long version)
Running time: 109 mins
Friday 26/09/08
19.50

The Duchess
Running time: 110 min (Contains moderate sex)
Friday 26/09/08
19.20

The Women
Running time: 114 mins (Contains moderate sex references and soft drug use)
Friday 26/09/08
12.45   15.30   18.00   20.30

Rocknrolla
Running time: 114 mins
Friday 26/09/08
12.00   21.30

The Boy In The Striped Pyjamas
Running time: 94 mins (Contains scenes of holocaust threat and horror)
Friday 26/09/08
13.00   14.40   15.20   2010

Disaster Movie
Running time: 87 mins   (Contains hard drug references, bleeped strong language and sex references)
Friday 26/09/08
11.15   13.15   15.15   17.15

The Strangers
Running time: 85 mins
Friday 26/09/08
19.40   21.55

Death Race
Running time: 105 mins
Friday 26/09/08
13.00   15.30   18.30   21.00

Redbelt
Running time: 99 mins
Friday 26/09/08
11.40   14.00   16.45   19.00   21.40

Righteous Kill
Running time: 101 mins
Friday 26/09/08
13.00   15.15   17.50   20.30

Swing Vote
Running time: 120 mins (Contains one use of strong language)
Friday 26/09/08
14.20   17.10   20.00

Taken
Running time: 94 mins
Friday 26/09/08
13.30   16.00   18.20   20.45

PIZZA KITCHEN

If it's the ultimate pizza you want,
Pizza Kitchen in Vivelchester city centre,
Vivel Square is the only place to be.
Offering you great deals all year round.

Opening hours

Monday to Friday	11:30–23:00
Saturday	11:00–24:00
Sunday	11:30–23:00

Part B: Activity answers and solutions

Budgeting answers

Prioritising activity 1 answers

Taxi driver Jack's budget sheet

1   Mortgage

2   Council tax

3   Fuel bills, gas and electricity

4   Water rates

5   Repayment of personal loan

6   Phone bill

7   Food and groceries

8   Petrol

9   Garage fees for repairs to car

10   Expenditure for family (clothes etc)

11   Leisure (cinema, restaurants)

12   Holiday

13   Monthly motoring magazine

14   New fishing equipment

15   CDs for in-car player

Routledge
Taylor & Francis Group

Prioritising activity 2 answers

Nurses' budget sheet

1 Rent

2 Council tax

3 Electricity

4 Food

5 Phone bill

6 Petrol

7 Car tyres

8 Shoes

9 Clubbing

10 Parties

11 Gown hire

12 Wine making kit

13 Jane's cookery classes

14 Karen's archery club

15 Denise's flying lessons

Prioritising activity 3 answers

Brian's budget sheet

1 Gas and electricity

2 Food

3 Clothing

4 Petrol

5 Toiletries

6 Household cleaning products

7 Newspapers

8 Weekly football magazine

9 Night out (cinema, pub)

10 Holidays

11 Tickets for football match

12 Paint balling sessions

13 Take-away food

Routledge
Taylor & Francis Group

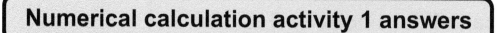

Numerical calculation activity 1 answers

Mrs Higgins' budget sheet

Incoming:	Salary =	£400.00
	Child benefit =	£31.00
	Total =	**£431.00**

Outgoing:	
Mortgage	£105.00
Council tax	£10.00
Gas and electric	£30.00
Food	£70.00
Childcare	£40.00
Petrol	£30.00
Mobile phone bill	£25.00
Clothes	£25.00
Total =	**£335.00**

Mrs Higgins can do without these items each week:

Magazines	£10.00
Lottery	£5.00
Cinema	£20.00
Plants	£15.00

Without these non-essential items, Mrs Higgins can save a total of £50.00 per week towards her holiday.

Routledge
Taylor & Francis Group

Numerical calculation activity 2 answers

Kevin's budget sheet

Incoming:	Salary =	£350.00
	Total =	**£350.00**

Outgoing:	
Rent and council tax	£125.00
Electricity	£14.00
Food	£50.00
Phone bill	£15.00
Petrol	£36.00
Car insurance	£5.00
Life insurance policy	£4.00
Total =	**£249.00**

Kevin can do without these items each week:

CDs	£8.00
Gym session	£10.00
Cinema and pub	£30.00
Magazines	£8.00

Without these non-essential items, Kevin can save a total of £56 per week towards a new car.

Routledge
Taylor & Francis Group

Numerical calculation activity 3 answers

Kate's budget sheet

Incoming:	Jobseeker's allowance =	£47.95
	Total =	£47.95

Outgoing:	
Board money to parents	£15.00
Mobile phone	£5.00
Bus fares	£7.00
Make-up	£6.00
Clothes	£10.00
Total =	£43.00

Kate can do without these items each week:

Fashion magazine £5.00

Cinema £10.00

As shown above, Kate could also reduce her spending on clothes from £20 to £10 a week, to make an additional saving. Without these non-essential items, Kate can save a total of £25 per week.

Routledge
Taylor & Francis Group

Bill terminology answers

Bank statement terminology: Activity 1 answers

Bank statement terminology

1 A document giving you information about your bank account.

Bank statement

2 Funds paid into your bank account.

Deposit

3 Allowing a debit as regular payment to a company for a service provided eg a phone bill.

Direct debit

4 Funds taken out of your bank account.

Withdrawals

5 Allowing your bank to pay money from your account on a regular basis to an external party.

Standing order

6 How much money you have in your account.

Balance

7 Your personal number.

Account number

8 Number of a particular branch.

Sort code

Living with an Acquired Brain Injury — This page may be photocopied for instructional use only. © Nick Hedley 2011 — Routledge Taylor & Francis Group

Bank statement terminology: Activity 2 answers

Calculate answers to the questions and write them in the boxes provided.

1 What is the total of the two lowest withdrawals from 03/08/09 to 31/08/09?

£23.23

2 What was the total amount of money paid into Ms Smith's account?

£160.00

3 What is the total amount of money withdrawn from a cash machine from 03/08/09 to 31/08/09?

£30.00

4 How many times did Ms Smith use her debit card from 03/08/09 to 31/08/09?

3 times

5 Look at the end balance on Ms Smith's bank statement. Is her account in credit or debit?

Credit

6 How much disability living allowance (DLA) was paid into her account between 03/08/09 and 31/08/09?

£95.00

7 How much money was withdrawn from Ms Smith's bank account between 03/08/09 and 31/08/09?

£181.26

8 How many times was money taken out of Ms Smith's bank account in the period of time covered by the statement?

7 times

Council tax bill terminology answers

Write the answers to the questions in the boxes provided.

1 Date the bill was issued.

> **Date of issue**

2 Details of how the money from your council tax is spent.

> **Details of charge**

3 The personal number you will need if you contact the council about your bill.

> **Reference number**

4 The dates you are being billed for.

> **Charge for period**

5 Bill paid once a year.

> **Annual**

6 The amount of council tax you must pay now.

> **Amount due**

7 Name another way that you could pay your council tax so you would not have to pay in one large amount.

> **Instalments**

8 Which service receives the least amount of council tax funds?

> **Fire and rescue**

Routledge Taylor & Francis Group

Home phone bill terminology answers

These questions are about the phone bill you have been given. In the cost of calls summary:

1 How many free calls were made? | **3**

2 How long did they last? | **30 minutes, 21 seconds**

3 How much did they cost? | **£0.00**

4 How many daytime calls were made? | **115**

5 How long did they last? | **4 hours, 19 minutes, 22 seconds**

6 How much did they cost? | **£14.91**

7 How many evening and weekend calls were made? | **18**

8 How long did they last? | **2 hours, 25 seconds**

9 How much did they cost? | **77p**

10 What was the total cost of calls? | **£15.69**

11 How much were the benefits? | **£1.29**

12 How much were the rental charges? | **£91.15**

13 How much was brought forward? | **£2.55**

14 How much VAT was added to the bill? | **£20.52**

15 How much do you have to pay Maximal Telecom? | **£28.62**

Mobile phone bill terminology answers

1 Number you must quote when making enquiries about your bill.

Account number

2 Fixed cost for your telephone line and any optional equipment.

Service charge

3 Number the bill is made out to.

Phone number

4 Tax added to your bill.

Value added tax or VAT

5 The personal plan you chose for your phone.

Price plan

6 Bill paid directly from your bank.

Direct debit

7 Charges made for your calls.

Usage charges

8 Money you pay to cover loss or damage to your phone.

Insurance

 Routledge Taylor & Francis Group

Water bill terminology answers

1 Number you must quote when making a payment.

Customer reference number

2 The date the bill was issued.

Issue date

3 Money brought forward from last bill.

Balance of last bill issued

4 Money already paid if you pay your bill weekly.

Sum of payments received

5 The amount of water you have used and how much it costs.

Usage

6 What else is included in your water bill which you must pay for?

Sewerage

7 How is the water that you use measured?

Cubic metres

8 Why does it say on this bill 'THIS BILL IS FOR INFORMATION ONLY?'

Because it is paid weekly in instalments

9 How many cubic metres of water have been used?

57

10 Write down the reading dates.

18/03/2008   18/12/2007

Routledge
Taylor & Francis Group

Living with an Acquired Brain Injury

Water bill terminology answers cont'd

11 What was the date of the previous bill issued?

24/12/07

12 What was the balance brought forward from the previous bill?

£58.23

13 How much does one cubic metre of water cost?

85.39p

14 What is the total amount for the bill?

£53.06

15 How many instalments have been paid?

3

16 What is the total of the money paid in instalments?

£76.00

17 What is the issue date of this bill?

27/03/2008

18 What is the amount the water charges are fixed at per year?

£28.80

19 What is the amount the sewerage charges are fixed at per year?

£64.20

20 Write down the meter number and the meter size.

97M913920   15

Routledge
Taylor & Francis Group

Route orientation answers

Shopping list A answers

Write down the order in which you would visit the places on your list to complete your shopping in the shortest time possible.

Enter the MetroCentre at the blue quadrant, lower floor.

1	**Sports World, lower blue 23.**
2	**Gap, lower grey 4.**
3	**Greggs, lower red 29.**
4	**Town square.**
5	**Post Office, upper green 34.**

Exit the MetroCentre at the blue quadrant, lower floor.

(This is the quickest way to complete the task. Discussion can stem from choosing different routes and shops.)

Routledge
Taylor & Francis Group

Shopping list B answers

Write down the order in which you would visit the stores on your list to complete your shopping in the shortest possible time.

Enter the MetroCentre at the red quadrant, lower floor.

1	**Cash machine, lower red 42.**
2	**HMV, lower red 28.**
3	**Timpson, lower red 26.**
4	**Primark, lower red 16.**
5	**Clinton Cards, lower red 7.**

Exit the MetroCentre at the red quadrant, lower floor.

(This is the quickest way to complete the task. Discussion can stem from using alternative routes and shops.)

Living with an Acquired Brain Injury

R Routledge
Taylor & Francis Group

Shopping list C answers

Write down the order in which you would visit the stores on your list to complete your shopping in the shortest time possible.

Stores on two levels have in-store stairs, so you can use these.

Enter the MetroCentre at the blue quadrant, lower floor.

1	**Abbey Bank, upper green 1.**
2	**Post Office, upper green 34.**
3	**Top Man, upper green 7.**
4	**HMV, for DVD, upper red 40. Go downstairs in-store to**
5	**HMV, for music CD, lower red 28.**
6	**River Island, lower red 37.**
7	**Café Gio, lower green 33.**
8	**Boots, lower green 14.**
9	**WH Smith, lower green 28.**
10	**Marks & Spencer, lower green 1.**
11	**Mothercare, lower grey 1.**
12	**Mulroy Antiques, upper blue V6, in the blue village.**

Exit the MetroCentre at the blue quadrant, upper floor.

(This is the quickest way to complete the task. Discussion can stem from using alternative routes and shops.)

  Routledge
Taylor & Francis Group   Living with an Acquired Brain Injury   **105**

Shopping list D answers

Write down the order in which you would visit the stores on your list to complete your shopping in the shortest time possible.

Enter the MetroCentre at the blue quadrant, lower floor.

1   **Disney Store, lower grey 5.**

2   **T-Mobile Store, lower green 23.**

3   **Thorntons, lower green 17.**

4   **Tie Rack, lower green 8. Take the escalator to upper level.**

5   **Professional Cookware Company, upper red 53.**

6   **Model Zone, upper red 42.**

7   **Buffet King, upper red 25. Down escalator (yellow quadrant).**

8   **Parker Tools, lower yellow 24.**

9   **Collectables, lower yellow 15. Go up escalator (yellow quadrant).**

10   **Quickstitch, upper yellow 9.**

11   **EWM, upper blue 16.**

12   **Early Learning Centre, upper grey 2.**

13   **The Paper Mill Shop, upper grey 4.**

14   **Poundland, upper blue 6.**

Exit the MetroCentre at the blue quadrant, upper floor.

(This is the quickest way to complete the task. Discussion can stem from using alternative routes and shops.)

Routledge
Taylor & Francis Group

Planning a night's entertainment answers

24-hour clock activity answers

Bus leaves Coach Lane Campus at 19:56.

What time does it arrive at Cruddas Park?

24-hour clock 20:29   **12-hour clock** 8.29pm

Bus leaves Cochrane Park at 20:28.

What time does it arrive at Denton Burn?

24-hour clock 21:11   **12-hour clock** 9.11pm

Bus leaves Sandyford at 21:14.

What time does it arrive at Whickham View?

24-hour clock 21:39   **12-hour clock** 9.39pm

Bus leaves Chillingham Road shops at 21:33.

What time does it arrive at Scotswood?

24-hour clock 22:07   **12-hour clock** 10.07pm

Bus leaves Haymarket John Dobson Street at 22:02.

What time does it arrive at Slatyford?

24-hour clock 22:29   **12-hour clock** 10.29pm

Routledge
Taylor & Francis Group

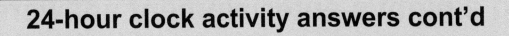

24-hour clock activity answers cont'd

What time is the last bus from Sandyford?

24-hour clock | 22:56   **12-hour clock** | 10.56pm

What time does the last bus arrive at Slatyford?

24-hour clock | 23:24   **12-hour clock** | 11:24pm

Routledge Taylor & Francis Group

Part C: Reusable resources

Payment taken Payment received Title	Money in	Money out	Resulting bank account balance

Budgeting table

Routledge
Taylor & Francis Group

Orientation street planner

1

2

3

4

5

6

7

8

9

10

11

12

13

14

15

16

17

18

19

20

Routledge
Taylor & Francis Group

Day/night out entertainment planning sheet

	Start:
	Arrive:

	Start:
	End:

	Start:
	End:

	Start:
	Return home:

 Routledge Taylor & Francis Group

Google earth and Google maps 'quick start' user guides

You must have an internet connection to use both pieces of this software.

Google earth

1 Type this internet address into your URL box at the top of your internet explorer software:
   http://www.google.co.uk/intl/en_uk/earth/index.html

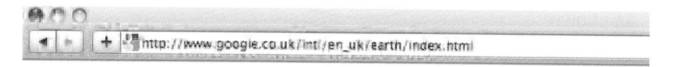

2 Push the 'enter' button on your keyboard. You should now be taken to the Google earth download website:

This website contains all the relevant instructions for using Google earth. However, this 'quick start' guide only gives you a brief, easy grasp of how the software works.

Click on 'Download Google earth' and this will take you to the next screen.

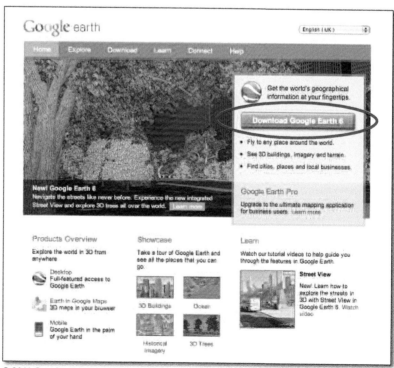

© 2011 Google

R Routledge
Taylor & Francis Group

Living with an Acquired Brain Injury

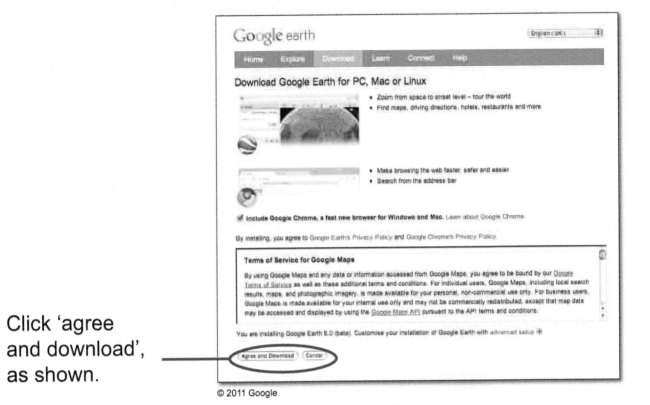

© 2011 Google

Click 'agree and download', as shown.

3 The Google earth installer software will then download to your PC. Go to this new icon (shown below) and double click on it.

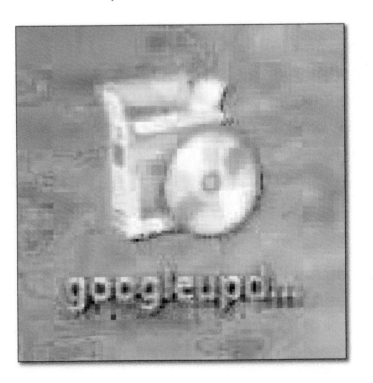

Routledge
Taylor & Francis Group

4 Another window pops up, showing the downloading process. When the colour bar is full, the window will disappear, and Google earth itself will start up, looking like this:

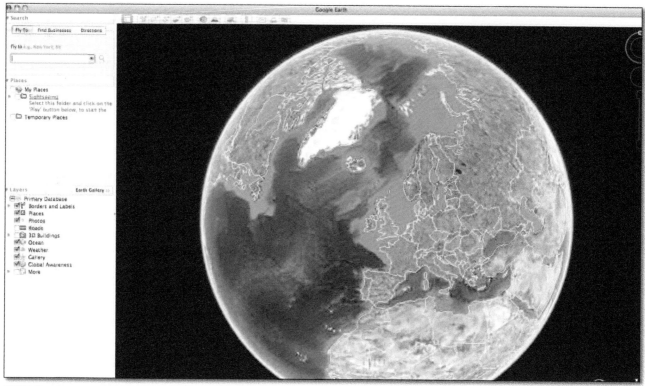

© 2011 Google

5 An image of the earth will appear. If you hold down the left button on the mouse, while moving the mouse over the map, you can drag to a specific location. Double click on the area that you want to look at and the view of the earth on the screen will zoom in. The various stages of this zoom function are displayed below.

A

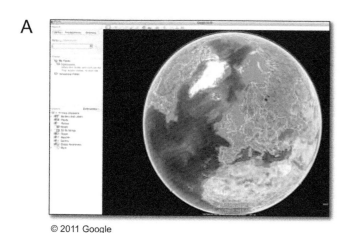

© 2011 Google

B

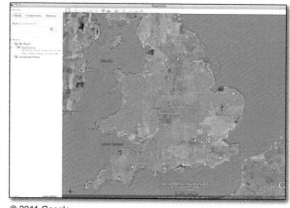

© 2011 Google

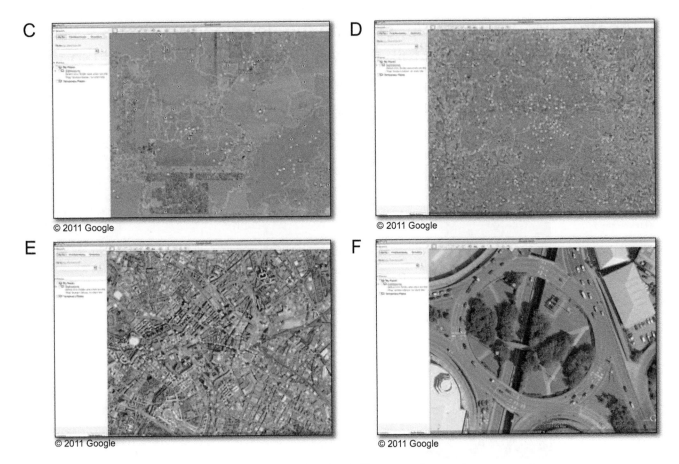

C © 2011 Google

D © 2011 Google

E © 2011 Google

F © 2011 Google

Google earth gives a photorealistic 3D overhead map view.

6 On the left of the screen is a grey panel, circled here:

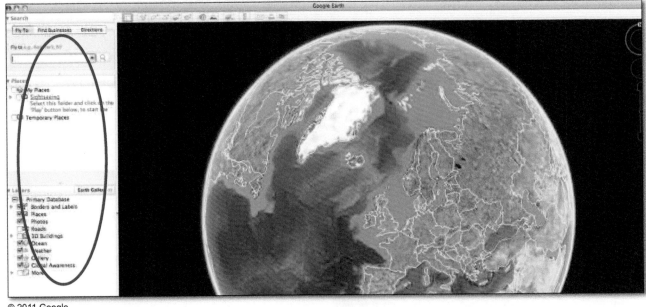

© 2011 Google

Routledge
Taylor & Francis Group

7 The grey panel is where you enter information, ie the places you would like to see on Google earth.

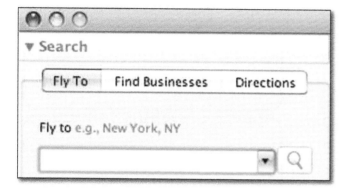

Near the upper part of the grey panel there are three headings/tabs. Click on the one you want to use. The first one is 'Fly To', the second is 'Find Business' and the third is 'Directions'.

Fly To

Click on the circled heading 'Fly To' at the top of the information bar. A box appears in which you type the name of the place you wish to see a map of. As an example, I have used the general place name 'hospital'. When the magnifying glass icon (the search button) is clicked, a series of results will appear in the largest circled box. As there are many hospitals in the country, a list of them is displayed. Below each name is the corresponding area, town or city, so that you can identify the particular hospital you are looking for.

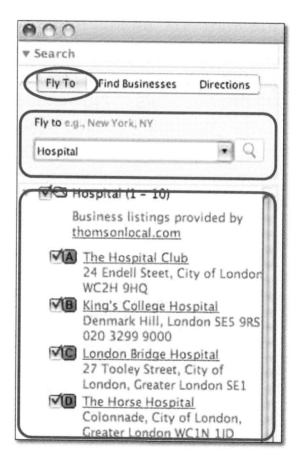

By double clicking on the name of the particular hospital you are looking for in this box, the map view will find its exact location and zoom in on it. From this point on, you can then choose to pull back slightly, or a great deal, and see the larger area, ie a map of your 'destination'.

HOT TIP If you know the postcode of the place you are searching for, write it in the search boxes used in Google. This makes the process quicker. Using postcodes is far more accurate than words or street names.

Find Businesses

There are two boxes below the heading 'Find Businesses' which enable you to do just that. The first box is for the name of the business you wish to search for (eg, again I have used the word or 'business', so 'Hospital'). The second box is for the town or city the business is in (in this case, Newcastle upon Tyne). Again, in the third box, search results (which are displayed when you click the magnifying glass icon) provide a list of all the hospitals in Newcastle upon Tyne. As above, double click on the hospital you were looking for, and the map will zoom in for you.

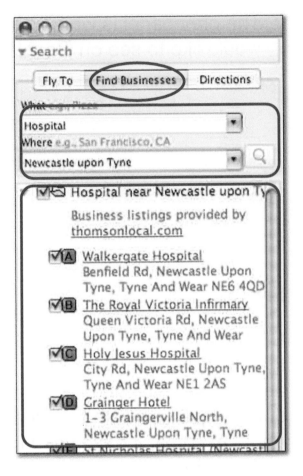

Directions

There are another two boxes under the third heading 'Directions' (circled at the top of the bar). However, they have different purposes from the boxes in the other headings. The first box is entitled 'From', and the second is 'To'. The 'From' box is where your journey starts, and the 'To' box is where you are going, your destination.

Under the 'Directions' heading, the search results in the large box entitled 'Printable view', is your journey plotted in stages, from where you begin, to your destination.

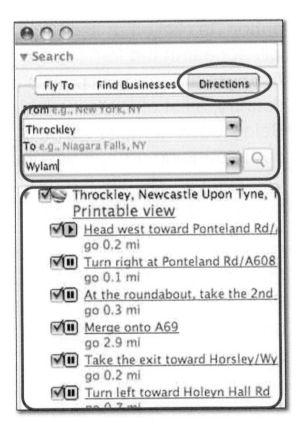

R Routledge
Taylor & Francis Group

Double click on any of these and you will be shown a closer look at that particular part of your journey. You will find the results of the queried journey from A to B are also shown on your map. You can print this out and take it on your journey.

8   There is another icon bar, above the map on Google earth. It looks like this:

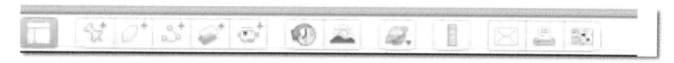

To find out what each icon does, hold the cursor over the icon for a few seconds and a small label appears which tells you the function.

In this 'quick start' guide you can manage without using most of the icons on the bar. However, a really useful icon is the last one on the right. You can click on this icon to convert the Google maps 2D image into a Google earth 3D map image. To the left of this icon is the printer icon symbol. This is used to print out your map. When the print window appears you will be given a variety of options. Choose how you would like the map of Google earth to be presented.

9   This journey plotted and shown on the map, as a purple line, is displayed below:

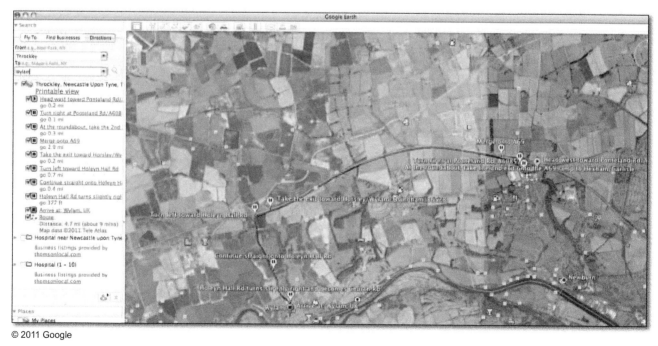

© 2011 Google

Routledge
Taylor & Francis Group

10 All software of this nature has its negative points, or issues that newer software improves upon. Google earth, being such a good visual representation of a place, does not use actual street names in most cases (see picture). Street names can be helpful and are used for the street planner sheets provided in this book. However, streets can appear far different when you are walking through them. Google maps does include most street names and we will look at this now.

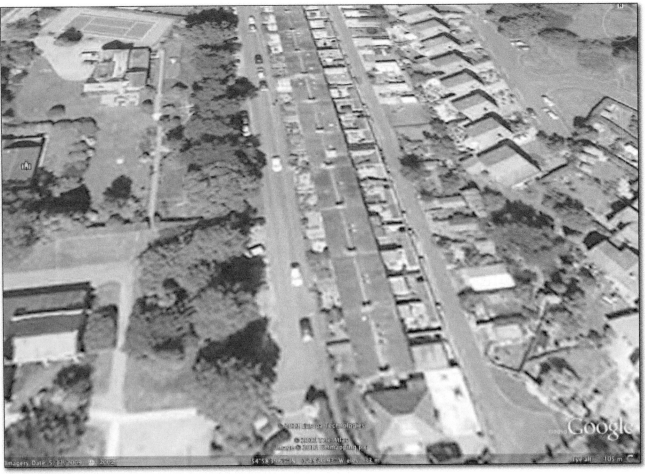

© 2011 Google

Routledge
Taylor & Francis Group

Google maps

1 Google maps is visually very similar to the A–Z. Unlike Google earth, downloading of the software to your PC is not necessary, as it is part of the online Google search engine and so is always present. To find it, go to the Google search engine homepage and click on the word 'Maps', shown and circled in the screenshot below:

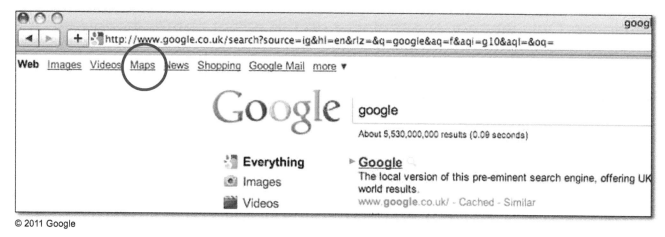

© 2011 Google

You will then be taken to a page like the one shown below:

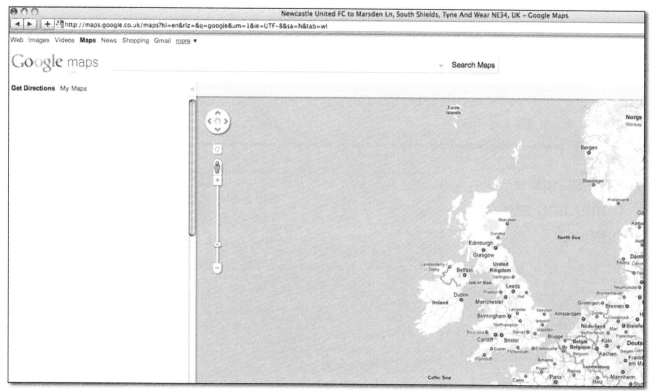

© 2011 Google

Routledge
Taylor & Francis Group   Living with an Acquired Brain Injury

2 The controls and icons for Google maps are very similar to Google earth. Google maps does, however, show street names, which is particularly beneficial in route orientation. Google maps will be perfect for use with the orientation street planner sheets provided with this book, to photocopy from part C, or print from the CD provided. From a long distance, as demonstrated by the Google maps screenshot on the previous page, street names cannot be seen at first. Use the same method of zooming into the map as with Google earth, double clicking on the area you want to see closer. Only when you get closer do the street names become clear. Here is an example of this:

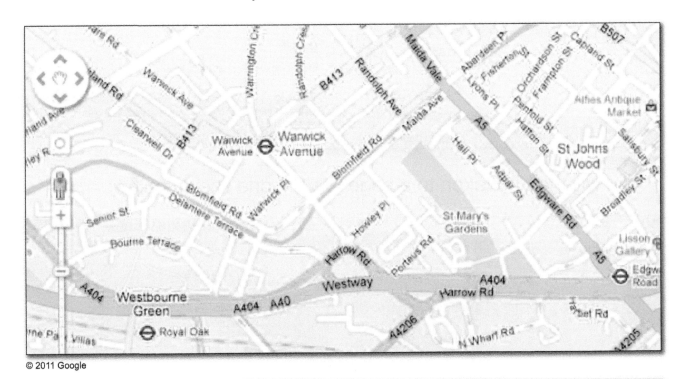

© 2011 Google

Closer-up (including street names):

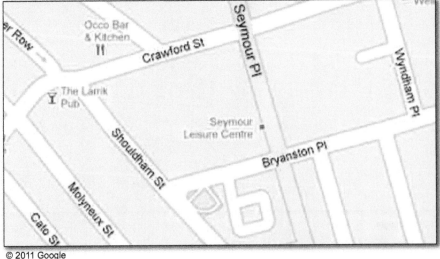

© 2011 Google

Routledge Taylor & Francis Group

3 On the left of the Google maps screen is another bar with icons and text. The Google maps bar has two different headings that can be clicked on. This is a 'quick start guide', and only gives the information you need to get started. The heading 'Get Directions' (as circled) is of most interest for swift use in terms of route orientation.

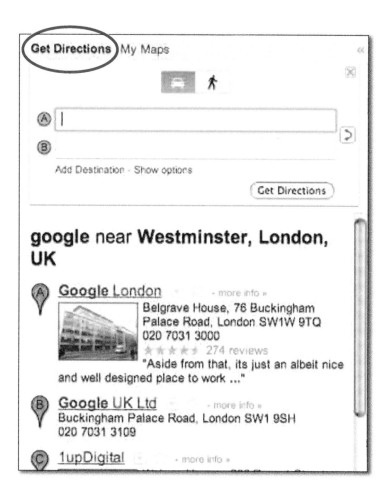

It works in the same way as the 'Directions' part of Google earth. Here, the two boxes are entitled A and B. This is a reference to the phrase 'getting from A to B', where A is your starting point and B is your destination.

You type in the 'From' box where you are leaving to begin your journey or trip (your house or where you are usually located), and then type in the 'To' box where you are going (your destination).

4 Click on 'Get Directions', and you will see a blue line; showing the place you are starting out from (A) and the route to your destination (B). In the large box below the A and B boxes, after clicking 'Get Directions', you will be given a series of stages of the journey, including the time it will take, on average, to reach that stage. Please be aware, however, that these suggested journey duration times are based on road travel while in a vehicle. An example of this is shown below, including the completed A and B boxes:

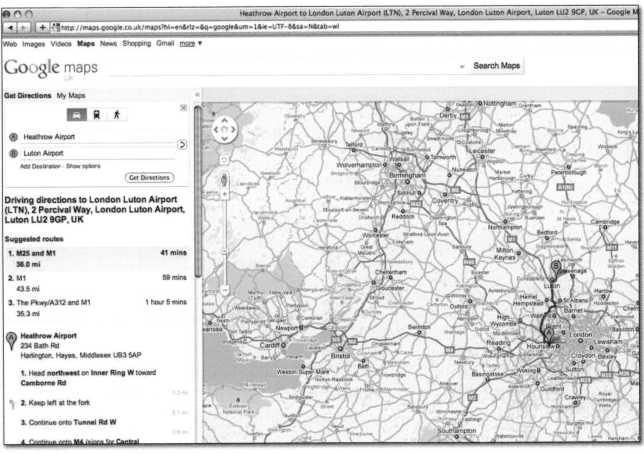

© 2011 Google

Routledge
Taylor & Francis Group

Google maps

5 As with Google earth, it is possible to zoom in on the view of the map to get closer to your planned journey route. With Google earth, we are given a photorealistic map image, which often shows you that it is not a good option to walk some parts of the suggested journey route. Google maps does warn of this, and often the map route planner may suggest walking through a river! The search icon it is best to click to obtain walking directions is circled in the screenshot below. Also circled is a Google maps warning.

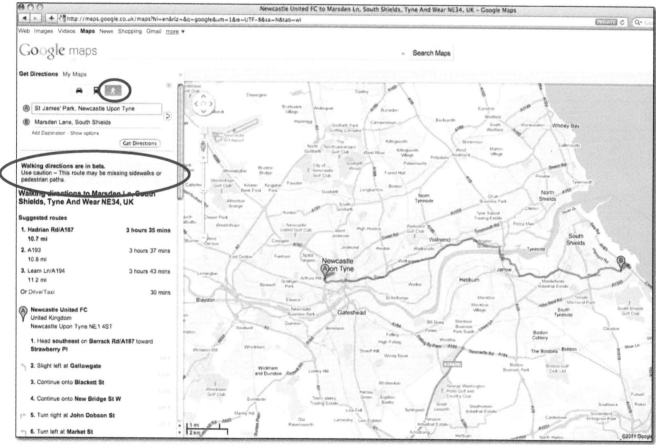

© 2011 Google

Routledge
Taylor & Francis Group

Living with an Acquired Brain Injury

6 Using a combination of the two formats of Google earth and Google maps can be beneficial in planning your journey. Earlier, in the Google earth map guide, we showed an icon to click on if you want to see the same route on Google maps. Below shows another icon in the top right of the Google map (circled), which performs a similar function; turning the Google map version into a Google earth map:

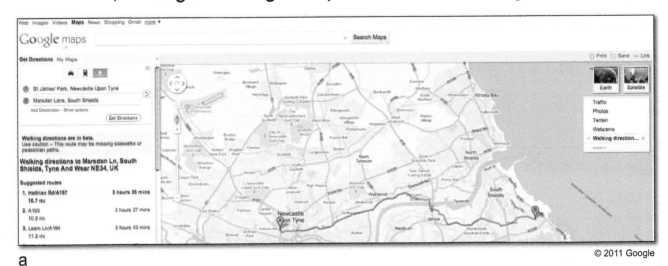

© 2011 Google

a

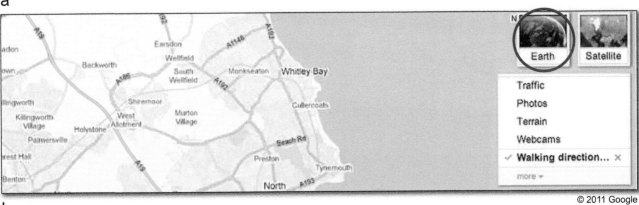

© 2011 Google

b

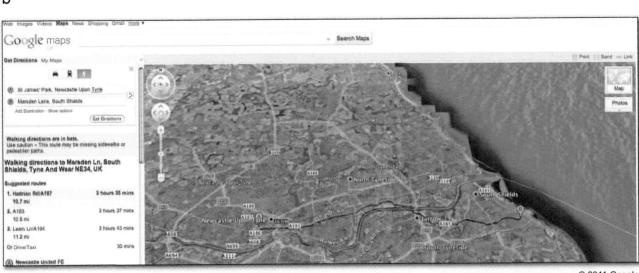

© 2011 Google

c

Routledge
Taylor & Francis Group

Final points to note

Despite the warnings issued in these 'quick start' guides concerning the negative points to watch out for, both pieces of software offer excellent possibilities in orientating yourself. The main focus for using these activities should encourage the idea of pre-planning, to ensure that any trips out go as smoothly as possible.

These maps, particularly Google maps (and the A–Z) will work well with the street planner sheet provided in this book and on the CD. The day/night out entertainment planning sheet could also be used for planning times and for remembering the things you need, not just for a night's entertainment. It can be seem as a list of 'things to do', with extra planning and memory aid.

Obviously, it may not always be practical to take so many sheets of paper out with you, but you can use these resources in advance of going out, and perhaps write down the important things to remember on a single sheet of paper, as a 'more structured' list of things to do, with times and directions, or street names included. Ultimately, safety should come first, and pre-planning can be one of the biggest advantages you will have when going out.

One point worth mentioning is the weather, which should always be taken into account. Very bad weather can majorly disrupt roads, pathways and public transport services. Luckily, in the UK, this type of weather is not common.

In terms of Google earth and maps, there are many other features available. As these are just 'quick start' guides, you have only been provided with the basics to get you started if you are unfamiliar with the software.

As previously mentioned, the website you download Google earth from contains many instructions about the various features the software offers. It is even possible to purchase an updated Google earth, which is in full 3D and has moving parts, sound effects and other features. Note that the Google earth covered in this guide is the free to download version.

For Product Safety Concerns and Information please contact our EU
representative GPSR@taylorandfrancis.com Taylor & Francis Verlag GmbH,
Kaufingerstraße 24, 80331 München, Germany

Printed and bound by CPI Group (UK) Ltd, Croydon, CR0 4YY
01/05/2025
01858600-0001